DRUGS
DEMONS
DOCTORS
and
DISEASE

"*To every thing there is a season, and a time to every purpose under the heaven:*

A time to be born, and a time to die; a time to plant and a time to pluck up that which is planted; A time to kill, and a time to heal; a time to break down, and a time to build up;"

ECCLESIASTES 5:1-3

DRUGS
DEMONS
DOCTORS
and
DISEASE

By

PERRY A. SPERBER, M.D.
Daytona Beach, Florida

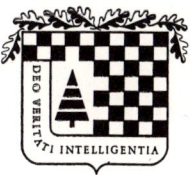

WARREN H. GREEN, INC.
St. Louis, Missouri, U.S.A.

Published by
WARREN H. GREEN, INC.
10 South Brentwood Blvd.
St. Louis, Missouri 63105, U.S.A.

All rights reserved

© 1973 by WARREN H. GREEN, INC.
Library of Congress Catalog Card No. 70-111808

Printed in the United States of America
(185)

DEDICATION

This book is affectionately dedicated to my wife Muriel, my daughters Gayle and Carol, and granddaughter Debbie; to my **sons** *Perry, Tom, and grandson Bryan.*

ACKNOWLEDGMENTS

I wish to acknowledge the help I have received in writing this book from my wife Muriel, my daughter Gayle Freeman, and my assistant Ethel Howard. I want to especially thank Ethel Howard for typing the manuscript and Librarian Alice Duva for helping me to procure research material for the book.

P.A.S.

INTRODUCTION

THE PURPOSE OF THIS BOOK is to give the non-professional individual an insight into the complex world of drugs.

To understand how we arrived at our present stage of knowledge, one must know the history of man and drug, for these two have been intimate friends long before recorded history.

In following the story of medicine, we are also pursuing the romantic saga of drugs. This book, accordingly, becomes a history of medicine and an anthology on drugs.

Our work is not intended to be a do-it-yourself kit for the non-professional person. For this reason, no dosages have been given for the administration of any drugs. The physician is the only one qualified and trained to prescribe medications. He is constantly studying and upgrading himself on drug usage, drug antagonism, drug interaction, drug abuse and other pertinent facts related to his profession.

The physician should be the final arbiter in deciding when, how, and what to prescribe for treating various disorders. There is an old aphorism in medicine which says that he who has himself for a physician has a fool for a doctor.

As modern technology moves ahead, rapid advances are being made in unraveling the causes of disease and the means to prevent or cure them. An exciting future is coming into sharp focus as the struggle to halt disease, advance health measures, retard the aging processes, limit population, and control pollution looms near.

CONTENTS

	Page
INTRODUCTION	vii
ACKNOWLEDGMENTS	ix

Chapter

		Page
I.	IN THE BEGINNING	3
II.	ANCIENT MEDICINE	17
III.	MEDIEVAL MEDICINE	49
IV.	SEVENTEENTH AND EIGHTEENTH CENTURY MEDICINE	57
V.	THE NINETEENTH CENTURY	73
VI.	THE TWENTIETH CENTURY	107
VII.	PREVENTIVE DRUGS	137
VIII.	DIAGNOSTIC DRUGS	141
IX.	SURGICAL DRUGS	147
X.	PSYCHIC DRUGS	155
XI.	RESPIRATORY TRACT, EYE AND CARDIOVASCULAR DRUGS	200
XII.	GASTROINTESTINAL DRUGS	213
XIII.	SKIN AND ALLERGY DRUGS	222
XIV.	ARTHRITIS DRUGS	230
XV.	URINARY TRACT DRUGS	235
XVI.	PARASITIC DRUGS	238
XVII.	CANCER DRUGS	242
XVIII.	DRUG INTERACTIONS	253
XIX.	DRUGS AND THE BIOLOGICAL TIME CLOCK	265
XX.	POLLUTION	281

DRUGS, DEMONS,

DOCTORS and DISEASE

Chapter One

IN THE BEGINNING

WHAT IS A DRUG? I am sure you will get many different answers from people, if you ask them this simple question.

Some will tell you that drugs are narcotic and psychedelic preparations. Others will say that drugs are medicines prescribed by doctors. A few may even state that a drug is something made by a druggist, although today a druggist compounds practically nothing, for almost everything he dispenses comes already prepared. The average individual does not consider as drugs such things as aspirin, laxatives, headache preparations, and vitamins.

Actually, what does the word "drug" mean? If we try to trace back its original meaning we run into a hangup. The word seems to have been derived from the French "drogue" and appears in old Middle English as "drogge." Around the 15th century, there seems to be a confusion in the manuscripts between "drogge" and dragge," the latter meaning dredge. Trying to probe back beyond this time leads to a dead end.

The word was certainly not Latin nor Greek in origin. A suggestion has been made that the word drug comes from "droge vate," a Low German term for dry vat, referring to dry casks in which drugs were stored. According to this theory, drug is derived from droge by error, referring to dry (vat) instead of the contents of the vats. In early modern English, the word drogge had become "drugg" or "drugge." From here it was just a short step to "drug."

Drugs, Demons, Doctors, and Disease

How do we define the word drug? One dictionary states that any substance used in medicine is a drug; formerly the term was used, and is still used by the French, to include all ingredients used in chemical, pharmaceutical, and dyeing procedures, as well as in the arts. Another dictionary says that a drug is a narcotic or poisonous preparation, as well as a substance used to prevent or cure disease or improve mental or physical health. Still another dictionary defines drug as any animal, mineral, or vegetable substance used in the preparation or composition of medicines, also any ingredient used in chemical preparations in the arts. We shall take a broad view of the term drug and develop this concept as we go along.

The legal dispenser or handler of drugs is known as a **druggist** or a pharmacist. We know the derivation of the latter word, for it comes from the Greek and has a most interesting connotation. The Hellenic word "pharmakeia" means the use of drugs, potions, or spells. Hence, we are dealing with poisoning, witchcraft, or sorcery. A "pharmakeus" is one who prepares or dispenses drugs or poisons, therefore a poisoner, witch, or sorcerer. A "pharmakon" is a drug, medicine, or remedy. In Latin, "medicamentum" is the word for drug, and a druggist is a "medicamentarius." How did the use of drugs ever get started? We do not really know, but we surmise that in the beginnings of what were the original men from whom we descended, that they had already begun to know the difference between poisonous and non-poisonous fruits and plants. No doubt, they had gained some knowledge from the early ape-men or man-apes which had preceded them. But! Man is an experimental animal, and those who tasted of the unknown or tried the new, either made novel discoveries, got awfully sick, or lost their lives. Such is the progress of knowledge!

Prehistoric man, we may assume, was probably not much different from the primitive man encountered today or during recorded history He was a savage creature living primarily by his animal instincts. He killed for food and fought off his enemies with stones, stone weapons or sticks. He raped his women, hid in caves, and lit fires to keep off human and animal predators, wore animal skins and primitive adornments.

Early man, like animals, had some knowledge of self-care. Perhaps he had learned from them. A dog, for instance, licks his

4

wounds, limps on three legs when one is injured, scratches and bites his skin in trying to rid it of parasites. He exercises, stretches and relaxes in the sun. When sick, he seeks out and eats certain herbs and grasses to cause vomiting or laxative action.

Early man had acquired some instinctive knowledge of self-care from his anthropoid ancestors. He used such simple measures as licking wounds, biting, rubbing, and scratching his skin. He moistened wounds with saliva, soaked swollen areas, and applied leaves to cool an inflamed wound or first crushed the leaves and then immersed them in water before application. Are we today so far apart from our early ancestors? Not really!

Later on, as he and his companions learned to bind up one another's wounds and set fractured bones, one who excelled in this experience became the "physician" for the group. It is believed by most anthropologists that women were the first to attend the sick and this was especially true in labor where midwives took over.

Primitive men made certain drug discoveries which are quite remarkable. The South American Indian, for example, somehow stumbled on the drug Quinine found in the bark of the cinchona tree and used it to treat malaria, a use still prevalent today. A Spanish priest took the remedy back to Europe. How did the Indian discover the drug and its usage? It would be interesting to know. We might also ask how another Indian in South America found out that the extract from a certain vine, which we now know as Curare, when placed on an arrow or spear and shot into a human or animal, would paralyze and finally kill the recipient? This drug paralyzes the muscles of respiration and the victim asphyxiates very quickly. Therefore, the Indian does not have to trail a wounded animal very far. In modern medicine, Curare is used discreetly to relieve muscle spasticity during anaesthesia. We shall say more later about the discoveries of drugs made by primitive men.

Life and disease have probably coexisted since early times. Shortly after the creation of a species, it was undoubtedly soon attacked by some kind of disease. We know definitely that disease existed millions of years before man appeared on this earth. Streptococci germs have been found in Montana rocks over thirty million years old. Evidence of parasites in fossils over twenty-six million years old have been discovered. The most ancient finding so far has been a bacteria-like cell over three and a half billion years old that was found in Africa.

Drugs, Demons, Doctors, and Disease

The common diseases of plants, fish, insects, and mammals, we suspect, started soon after they were created. They began to suffer from infections, epidemics, pests, and other disorders. The evolution of organic life was accompanied by constant warfare with infecting organisms. According to Metchnikoff, disease and infection appeared on this earth in very remote times. He believed that disease began as an antagonism between two forms of life. Primitive cells battled each other for survival and often devoured one another. Metchnikoff called attention to epidemics occurring among the ancient amebas. He believed that viruses and bacteria early in the history of life became pathological or disease producers. Parasites began to infest living forms.

The fossilized bones of ancient animals gives us some medical history of the past. For example, there is evidence of bone infection, arthritis, and dental decay among dinosaurs. Renault has found various bacteria, such as micrococci and diplococci, in fossilized fish and other vertebrates that lived in the carboniferous age. There were insect and animal carriers, too, in those long-ago ages before man arose on earth. Monkeys and anthropoids had parasitic infections and so did early man. Even modern man is not immune and he suffers from worm, fluke, and other infestors. Arthritis has been discovered in ancient and modern mammals, the great apes, and modern man. Evidence of tuberculosis has been disclosed in ancient man, and the possibility of syphilis has been considered by some authorities.

Unfortunately, due to bodily decay, organic disorders and certainly functional disorders cannot be ascertained from fossilized remains. But we can remedy this by studying living anthropoids whose maladies have presumably not changed much in millions of years. Another source of information is the study of disease in primitive peoples who are living much like their ancestors, and knowledge gained from the past discloses primitive illnesses in historic records. From all these studies, we have gained a pretty good idea of the diseases afflicting primitive and prehistoric man.

From anthropology and paleontology, we know that certain races of early men and various species of animals became extinct. Why, we do not know! It is believed that violent and vicious plagues raged from time to time among prehistoric man, and probably also among animals, and could have been responsible for their disappearance. At least, it is one possible reason . . . and a good one.

Drugs, Demons, Doctors, and Disease

In the *history* of man, there is much evidence of the disappearance of racial groups due to pestilence. This was also unquestionably true in *prehistoric* epochs.

There are certain disorders which afflict modern man and animals today, and we have good reason to believe that they also existed among early man, and also were prevalent long before even the anthropoids were created. Such conditions are hereditary disorders and diseases due to viruses, bacteria, protozoa, metazoa, endocrine imbalances, congenital defects, dietary deficiencies, inborn errors of metabolism, and cancer. An erroneous opinion has existed that disease came into the world with man and is due to man's sinfulness. No doubt sin adds to man's woes, but diseases existed long before he got here.

When men first made a concerted effort to have one of their number assume the care of the injured and sick, we do not know. Probably, it was the Australopithecines, perhaps well over a million years ago. From what we actually know now, Cro-Magnon man, who appeared about thirty-five thousand years ago, has left the first record in history. One of their paintings found in France in the cave of the Three Brothers shows a man who is a medicine man, shaman, or sorcerer, quite similar in appearance to the medicine man of primitive tribes.

The job of medicine men has always been to appease the spirits which tormented the patients. Whatever he does, whether it be incantations, amputation of a finger, cauterizing a wound, burrowing a hole in the skull in the act of trephining, or performing a circumcision, he does for one purpose only. That is, to allow, force, or persuade an evil spirit to leave the body. Strange to say, all primitive medical folklore is based upon this principle of animism, the idea that the whole world is full of demons and that they are the prime cause of disease. The shaman, medicine man, or witch doctor employs magic to drive them out. In this demonic concept, medicine and surgery had their beginnings. Primitive man's conception of spirits preceded his development of divinities, which he later used for protection against evil demons.

The question that comes to mind now is, how did man conceive of demons and spirits? To understand this thinking, we must place ourselves in the world of primitive man and see his bewilderment at the forces of nature. What we consider normal and natural was for him the supernatural. The flash of lightening and the crash of thunder terrified him even as it does so many "moderns" today. For, he did not know what caused them. Modern man, knowing, still fears them. Puzzling to primitive man were the winds, rustling of leaves, fire, sunlight, moonlight, the stars, clouds, storms, rain, eclipses, earthquakes, echoes, flowing water, a churning lake, the sea, a shadow, pregnancy, birth, disease, death.

In view of the above, it was quite easy to imagine something alive and responsible for all this activity. For example, the primitive could see his own reflection in the water which moved with and mimicked his actions, and he could consider it his alter ego. He saw his shadow, just as he saw the shadows of his fellow men. It followed him wherever he went and the shadows of his companions did likewise for them. They could all walk through their companion's shadow and never feel anything. The most obvious conclusion was that is was a spirit being from another world and a being from which he could not escape. It was best to keep it happy.

Then, there was the dream world. It has always mystified mankind, and even does today. Sometimes a man dreams and when it is over, it is very hard for him to decide whether he was dreaming or whether it was true. How much more mystifying it must have been for an ignorant savage! Dreams can be quite frightening as we all know, so how did the primitive interpret them? Or, for that matter, any dream? Even twentieth century man often implies an import to it. The savage mind was sure he had seen spirits for how else could he interpret reflections, shadows, and the fearful reality of dream episodes. The world of spirits was very real indeed to early man. He did not doubt it at all.

He feared the spirits, for it is only natural to fear the unknown and unknowledgeable. He therefore tried to appease the supernatural and began to worship the spirits of the sun, moon, stars, winds, rivers, springs, trees, animals, and just about everything that had motion. After a while, instead of worshiping the object itself, he began to make representations of it by carvings of wood, bone, or stone, or even a mannequin-type simulation by using skins over wood, bone, or stone. Man thus passed from nature worship to fetish worship and venerated the symbol instead of reality and attributed to it the supernatural power.

Understanding disease even less than he understood his supernatural world, primitive man began to feel that such doings must be the work of a spirit, most likely an evil spirit, certainly not a good spirit. This was a logical conclusion in a world swarming with spirits. To get rid of a disease one must, therefore, in some way appease the demon, possibly with a sacrifice or a burnt offering. After all, when we look at the situation, what did a savage actually have to offer anyway in material goods?

A second concept of disease developed after some period of time. This was a new belief that, in addition to spirits, a human enemy could cause men to fall sick by putting a curse on them or getting a voodooist to do it, a belief still held today by many people. The human enemy would have to possess some supernatural power himself, or lacking it, invoke the help of a shaman who had such superpower. To neutralize this wickedness, one would need the help of a witch doctor who had counter spells or sorcery.

Later, a third idea evolved as to the cause of disease and this was based upon the thought that the spirits of the dead were offended by the living. These dead spirits could be those of men, animals, or even plants. It was easy to conceive of such beings, for certainly the dead went somewhere after they died and disintegrated. They obviously became spirits and you could certainly see them and converse with them in your dreams. Today, in the twentieth century, many people believe that the dead can come back to haunt them and inflict misfortune upon them. How many believe in the religion of spiritualism and in communication with the ghosts or souls of the dead? Very many indeed, and certainly very many more than will admit to it. So, how far are we really apart from our primitive ancestors? Despite technology, not really too much, I suspect.

To protect man from all the adversities which could be cast upon him by a swarming universe of spirits, a specialist was needed who understood and could deal with these powers. Such a man was the priest, medicine man, shaman, or magician. In primitive societies, one man usually combined all these offices. His function was to thwart the evils sent against his people. He had to deal with black magic which gave rise to disease, death, drought, famine, floods, devastating fires, and other natural disasters. White magic, which he invoked, was used to counteract these catastrophies and to produce rain when needed, to create fire as desired, to raise abundant crops, to provide good hunting, and to conquer disease, pestilence, and epidemics. He obviously was the man to provide the good life for his people—a life to which we moderns subscribe to and are still looking for. But our shamans have failed to provide it.

We have noted the primitive thinking of what causes disease, now we must come to the conception of how it takes place. There are three "hows." First, something enters the body. Secondly, something is absent from the body. Thirdly, a spell of sorcery strikes a part of the body or an object in close approximation to the body. The first theory is not too far off from the modern infectious and toxic theory of agents that can enter the body to produce sickness. Early man could not possess such knowledge and assumed a demon entered. The second theory of something being lacking in the body would correspond with our modern ideas of metabolic and deficiency diseases. As regards the third theory, modern psychiatry replaces the magic concept of exorcism and attempts to treat the affected psyche.

As we have pointed out, ancient man feared animals and worshiped them, for their strangeness mystified him. Even modern man and children are intrigued by animals in zoos, movies, and television. The cave paintings of Cro-Magnon men depicted many kinds of animals and also the witch doctor clad in an animal skin. His function here was probably to insure a good hunt, and then protect his people against the avenging demon spirits of the slain animals. Strange practices have evolved using animal skins. The ancient Gauls and Germans, along with the American Indians, wore animal skins to ward off evil spirits. The African wears a leopard skin or the mane of a lion. Teeth or bones of animals are worn as protective amulets by primitive tribesmen. The priests of Babylon conducted their rituals while dressed in fish skins. In ancient Ireland, a sick patient waited to get well, while being clad in the skin of a freshly sacrificed sheep.

Certain parts of animals, and humans too (for cannibalism has been a part of human experience), were considered specific for disease and were usually eaten raw. Among some savages consuming the whole body to heal sickness was an acceptable custom, at other times it was considered taboo. This was true among the ancient Germans, according to the historian Tacitus, and also occurred in the Roman and Greek sacrificial rituals to the underworld gods or spirits. Heart, liver, and brain were the most highly regarded organs, and blood itself was the best remedy. Scribonius Largus, a Roman physician, claimed the drinking of one's own blood was an effective remedy. These ancient beliefs were held and recorded even in the eighteenth century pharmacopoeias of useful drugs. In religious rituals, the belief of power in the blood carried over into sacrificial cakes or the sacrificial bread and wine.

While belief in the cause of disease as being due to evil spirits may sound ridiculous and superstitious to modern intelligent people, one must not be too critical of ancient man for his demonologic thinking. For this aborigine was looking for a reason and the demon idea looked as good as any to explain things. In any event, it was a beginning step on the long evolutionary road of medicine.

There are people in modern times who still cling to this most ancient supposition. For example, the Korean peasants believe that typhus, smallpox, and cholera devils roam through the air and can be scared and driven off by banging upon pots, pans, drums, and gongs. The Chinese peasants imagine that good and bad demons constantly swarm through the atmosphere. For some unknown reason, they have rationalized that good ones move in curves and bad ones in straight lines. For this reason, the Chinese have deliberately used curves in their architecture when they built houses, pagodas, and other types of buildings. In Polynesia, the natives feel that sacrifices must be rendered to those spirits of gods which bring about disease. The medicine given for the disorder is merely a vehicle through which the appeased one will put an end to the disorder.

Many of the practices of prehistoric folks were adopted by primitive tribes and have even survived to find their way into the cultures of modern civilized nations. Evidence of this is seen in modern steam baths and saunas. Massage is a direct hand-me-down from primitive steamings and massage. However, the purpose is somewhat different. The ancient idea was to exorcise the evil ones, while the modern thought is to "open the pores" and drive out the impurities from the body. Both concepts are wrong. The custom of kneading or pounding the body during massage had a definite design in the savage's mind. He was driving the demon towards the feet where he could escape, and so the direction of working was pedal. Another method of getting rid of a bad spirit was to cut the skin and let him flow out with the dripping blood. The above procedures eventually led to the development of what is known as Swedish massage and bloodletting.

Early man developed a knowledge of which organs were vital, such as the heart, lungs, and the liver. In his paleolithic paintings and sketches, this experience is portrayed in the kills. There is also evidence in these pictures of amputations of fingers, toes, eye gouging, castration, infibulation and other mutilations. Why? American Indians and African Bushmen cut off their fingers to get rid of demons of disease, or any attachment to death when burying a relative, or to avoid death when being near to a dying relative. By giving up a part of their person in the form of a digit, they believed they were ridding themselves of the evil spirit.

As a result of the spirit or demon psychology of prehistoric man, it was only natural for the early physicians to be magicians and their methods of treatment completely magic. Their prescribing of healing medications was wrapped in a mystic aura. The drugs had to be gathered at the most propitious time by the correct person using only special instruments while reciting magic incantations. This mystique had to take place when the sun or moon was in a very special phase in its course, or during the specific courses of the planets, plus a lot of other mumbo jumbo and hocus pocus. The esoterics conferred upon the medication a magic spell. To break the formalized procedure at any point would ruin the potency of the preparation. For, if all goes well, the patient will recover. If not, the doctor is responsible.

In most primitive cultures, a failure to cure is considered to be due to the power of superior magic being applied by a demon or enemy. Life and death in such societies are believed to be the result of the interaction of powerful forces, potent spirits, or other influences. The mightiest ones determine the present and the future.

Death, like disease, is due to mysterious or violent happenings. Neither was construed by the aboriginal mind as being a natural occurrence. On the contrary, death, like disease, was caused by demons, ghosts, or the action of medicine men. This conception, so universal among all primitive people, has led anthropologists to conclude that the ancestors of all of them had a common home at one time and in their subsequent wanderings carried with them this traditional belief.

The Babylonians believed that death arose as the result of a serpent tempting a woman to partake of a particular fruit in a garden which had been forbidden by a deity. In Genesis, we have a similar story which resulted in the downfall of man. Man, unable to explain death, supposed it was due to a wicked angel or the "angel of death." Certain African tribes felt that death resulted from one of their ancestors washing in a taboo river. The aborigines of Australia blamed a certain woman who ventured near a forbidden tree upon which a bat sat. As a result of this approach, the bat flew away and death was loosened upon the land. On and on the myths go.

Strange are the ways of man, and prehistoric man was no different in this respect than his descendents. Blood was red, therefore anything red resembled blood and had a life-giving quality. Such was the characteristic attributed to red earth. Cro-Magnon men covered their dead with red ochre to give them back a life-spirit. Various herbs were of value because of their color and each color contributed a quality. If a leaf resembled a certain organ, it was specific for treating the viscus. The location in which plants grew and their particular configuration gave them magical qualities. If a berry or fruit of a particular color or shape seemed to have cured a disease, then all berries of other plants of the same color or having leaves of a similar shape were curative also. In modern times, red meats and beets are believed to be blood building because of their red color.

Yet, superstition dies slowly, if ever at all. The folk mind of this and the last century produced some whoppers. Warts are caused by handling toads and can be cured by touching them with pebbles. Stump water cures freckles. Poor eyesight could be helped by bathing in water which had been touched by the red hot iron of the blacksmith. Enclosing a spider in a nutshell and wearing it about the neck cures malaria. A beetle in a bottle will cure whooping cough and, if this doesn't work, wrapping a spider in muslin and placing it on the mantel will do the job. If this also fails, riding on a bear, eating fried mice, or drinking owl broth are good remedies.

Among other gems are the following items: Venereal disease can be gotten rid of by giving it to a child or woman by contact. A child suffering from hernia can be cured by passing him through the fork in an ash tree. A tuberculous child can be cured by passing him through a woodbine wreath. One can get rid of rheumatism by crawling under a bramble bush. Hot mud packs and radioactive mud or water will cause arthritis to disappear. Sulfur and molasses will cure spring fever. Religious medals and amulets will ward off disease. If such ideas as we have mentioned, and there are many more than space will allow, can be believed in the nineteenth and twentieth century in highly civilized nations, how can we condemn primitive man who never had the educated chance to know better?

The study of the American Indians has given us an excellent insight into Stone Age medicine. The North, Central, and South American Indians had similar beliefs in their religious, medical, and cultural activities. They also had much in common with primitve peoples elsewhere. In religion, they were polytheistic. In medicine, they adhered to the demon theory of disease. They used drugs unknown to the European immigrants. Among these were balsam of Tolu, cascara, coca leaves (cocaine), capaiba, chenopodium, guaiac, curare, ipecac, sarsaparilla, jalap, quinine, and tobacco. These drugs provided emetic (vomiting) action, laxative purging, expectorant action, tonic stimulation, malaria relief, poisoning, worm killing, and local anesthesia.

The main source of primitive remedies came from the vegetable kingdom. Seeds, flowers, bark, limbs, leaves and roots provided the drugs. The Indians used yellow drugs to treat jaundice, red to make blood. Liverwort was given for liver disorders because its leaves were liver shaped, lungwort because it resembled the lungs, heart-shaped leaves were applied to the sore nursing breasts of women.

Tobacco was the Indians' sacred plant, and it was utilized in religious and magic rituals. It was chewed, along with coca leaves, to give the Indians hallucinations, in order to get themselves primed for talking to the Great Spirit. Tobacco was also thought to have many valuable qualities in combating all kinds of disease.

South American Indians concocted a number of intoxicating drinks. To make them more powerful they often added an extract from the poisonous plant datura. These drinks were used in ceremonial performances. The Indians, in addition, also took hallucinatory drugs. So did the Mexican Indians. They both used mescaline which comes from the button of the mescal cactus, psilocybin derived from a certain mushroom psilocybin mexicana, and dimethyl-tryptamine extracted from the bark of seeds of the mimosa tree. These psychedelic substances were employed in religious and healing rituals.

The North American Indians knew the properties of the red bean of Texas and the Peyote bean. The Kiowas used the red bean at meetings of their secret societies and enjoyed the delirious and narcotic effects of the bean. The Omahas preferred the peyote bean because of its pleasant feeling of abandonment and the beautiful colorful hallucinations.

For narcosis and pain relief, the Indians used datura, peyote, tzompatti, and a motor nerve paralyzer called thalcopolin.

Extracts of animal organs, bone, and ash, as well as blood and bile, were common medical remedies. Stones were also used such as jasper for treating hemorrhage and colic. Salt, gypsum, nitre, and saltpeter were utilized in medical therapy.

The most civilized Indians were the Mayans, Incas and Aztecs. Their medical and surgical skills were much superior to those of the primitive Indians. They knew how to set bones and encase them in plaster splints. They learned how to suture wounds with hair, to cauterize infected wounds, and to use ant heads as skin clips.

The Indians knew how to take enemas. They used animal bladders and forced water through a hollow turkey bone into the rectum. An animal bladder applied to a turkey quill was used as a syringe to irrigate an infected or dirty wound.

Among miscellaneous practices were bloodletting, cupping, and burning of incense on the skin, like the Chinese moxa procedure, to secure counter irritation. Some North American Indians immunized themselves against rattlesnake bite, which was quite frequent, by having themselves bitten by baby rattlers, and gradually using larger snakes until full grown snakes did the biting. Thus immunized they could stand occasional biting and suffer no reactions. The Indians also used primitive sauna baths. They made a house of animal skins airtight, then brought in hot stones and threw water upon them. It was a primitive sweatarium. Its purpose was to purify the body, propitiate evil spirits, and combat disease. Gradually, the sauna became a social gathering place.

Obstetrical practice was controlled by the women. Labor was short, rarely over three hours and attended with little pain. The position assumed by the woman in labor varied with the tribes. The Apache and Navaho used the half recumbent posture, the Crow knelt down, the Sioux delivered standing up, the Creeks lay on their stomachs with attached pillows and tightening straps. If labor was slow, the midwife, standing behind the woman, locked her hands over the abdomen and applied pressure; if not successful, a strap was tightened or the woman might be carried on her husband's back with her abdomen bumping against him. If none of these methods were successful, the midwife would insert her hand into the vagina or womb and tug on any presenting part available.

Abortion was seldom performed. Usually, if the father was a white man, it was permitted, for the Indians had no use for halfbreeds. Their procedures for doing abortions varied. In some tribes, walking on the woman's abdomen was the custom; in others a board was placed across the abdomen and rocked back and forth by two women seesawing. An internal method was the use of slippery elm, inserted into the neck of the womb, a method used in modern times by our own culture. The Indians occasionally employed what they considered abortion-producing medication. They prescribed extracts of pine bark, cedar, powdered rattlesnake, or bear claws. The value of such material is quite questionable.

When we look back at the medicine of the primitive man of the Stone Age, we were not too far ahead of him at the beginning of the twentieth century. However, in order to get to the great advances of our times, we must at this point move out of the Stone Age into recorded history and see the fascinating stories begin to unfold.

Chapter Two

ANCIENT MEDICINE

AMONG THE EARLIEST GREAT civilizations of which we are aware is that of the Sumerians. They were excellent craftsmen working with metals when the Egyptians were still in the stone age. According to Wooley, the excavator of the ancient city of Ur, the cities of Erech, Lagash, Kish, and Ur had well-organized governments and cultures around 5,000 B.C. Long before the biblical-mentioned city of Ur existed, a wealthy and highly cultured dynasty of kings ruled in the land of Sumer and Accad in the city of Kish, the most ancient city in this region.

Here, around 3000 B.C., were houses of brick with lavatories and bathrooms which had drains to carry off sewage into tanks located in the streets. From these subterranean containers, street cleaners removed the wastes. A tablet found in the city displayed a physician's personal seal. The Sumerians are credited by Langdon with inventing writing, He stated evidence of this was discovered in Kish about 4200 B.C. At first, it was picture writing, then became ideographic to express an idea. Later, it evolved into the cuneiform writing to express syllabic functions. The Babylonians, under their great king Hammurabi in the eighteenth century B.C., conquered the country. He formulated his famous law code which contains regulations for the practice of medicine. Our knowledge of these people and the Assyrians comes from their cuneiform writing on baked clay tablets.

Drugs, Demons, Doctors, and Disease

Early Babylonian medicine, like the Sumerian, had not progressed very far from primitive man's conception of demons and gods. Their medicine was strongly linked with religion and magic, all controlled by priests. In time, a guild of physicians and surgeons arose and practiced according to a code of definite rules. The priest-physician was given the name of "assipu," while the lay-physician was known as the "asu." The assipu treated internal and mental diseases. For these disorders were assumed to be caused by demonic action and therefore only amenable to religious and magic countermeasures. On the other hand, external conditions, which resulted in injury and violence to the individual, were considered to be the province of the asu who treated them with natural methods. The name asu was used like our common term doctor, but was also broadly applied to physician, seer, and scribe alike.

Hammurabi's code for medical practice ignored the assipu priest who had to contend with the punishment of men by gods, evil-demons, witches, unlucky stars, and the evil eye. Instead, it laid down laws for the asu practitioner who treated surgical cases where the cause of the affliction was known. Yet, the asu could not completely ignore the animistic medical beliefs of the masses of the people, and so he had to combine his natural methods with medication which had a tinge of magic and divination.

The healing god of Babylon was Ea, who was also god of the deep. He ruled the universe with Anu, god of heaven, and Bel, god of the earth. Ea was too mighty to be addressed directly for help, and so prayers went to his son Marduk to intercede for the petitioner. If a person was sick, relief was requested in the form of a charm or some special incantation. If the patient was under the spell of some witchcraft, a countermeasure was sought.

Associated with Marduk were city gods and also Ninib of Lagash who was the gods' own physician. Patron gods of the healing arts were Ninurta and his wife Gula. Their symbol was the serpent, adopted by the Greeks whom we will discuss later. In addition, there were gods of special disease syndromes and even a god for the physicians known as Ninazu. In order to properly help a patient, the priest had to call on the god who ruled over the particular disease.

After the gods came the despicable demons. There were seven major evil demons known as the maskims and also as the seven fiery phantoms. They opposed the works of the gods and were responsible for floods, earthquakes, tempests, and plagues.

After these major troublemakers came a host of minor demons which attacked man in every possible way. They assailed humans by ambush, and prepared various philters to get him in trouble, both morally and physically. They were devotees of the goddess Ishtar who presided over darkness and witchcraft, and who loved to seize victims at night and slay them, especially the young. Ishtar was feared by witches and also by streetwalkers who tried to placate her with various kinds of charms. Fear of demons was not peculiarly Babylonian, as we have said before, it was and still is universal in primitive societies and even in some modern cultures. The most feared of these demons were the horrible disease-producers such as Namtar and Dibbara, well known for causing pestilences.

If all these terrible creatures were not enough to make man's lot most miserable on earth, the Babylonians, in addition, believed in sorcerers who consorted with the powers of evil and forced men to do their will. As a result, the sorcerers acquired the ability to bring on sickness, death, and other horrible disasters. So great was their power, they could bring on disaster by a mere unpleasant look, speaking magic words, preparing potent drinks, and by the power inherent in the evil eye. Belief in the power of the evil eye occurred first in Babylonia where it was believed to cause disease. There are people even today who fear the consequences of gazing upon the evil eye, so strongly has this superstition been believed by people over the centuries.

The progress of medicine in Babylonia, Assyria, and Chaldea was impeded chiefly by the so-called science of astrology, which supported the idea that stars were divinities of supreme intelligence and ruled over the destinies of men, nations, and the universe. The popularity of astrology in these modern times attests to the universal, inherent power of superstition to firmly control the minds of men. To the ancient, every future earthly occurrence was wrapped up in the mystery of the stars and such events could only be read by the priests, and, today, of course, by the astrologers. These priests understood and spoke the language of the heavenly lights, knew the revelation of the gods, and therefore could, with great wisdom, predict the future of men, kings, and nations. Horoscopes were cast for individuals, just as in modern times. Astrological medicine determined the ancient's way of life, his culture, his health, his religion, his diseases, and the way he would die.

Primitive man venerated rivers and streams, and so did the Babylonians. Primitive man venerated the stars, and so did the Babylonians. To the latter they were gods. The astrologer, who communicated with these star-gods, could help a patient. All he needed to know was the graph of the zodiac, a knowledge of where the planets were on the day the patient was born, and the day he took sick. Hippocrates, the father of medicine, who was born many centuries later, adopted some of the Babylonian thinking. He said, "Attention must be paid to the rising of stars, especially Sirius and Arcturus, and to the setting of the Pleiades. For most diseases reach a crisis during such periods." He further stated that astronomy is of great importance in the practice of medicine.

Astrology had a stranglehold on medicine well into the eighteenth century. Physicians strongly believed in astrologic diagnoses and astrologic remedies. Traditionally, over the centuries, medical astrology was supported by the leading physicians in all countries. Astrologists have even claimed that Hippocrates was the first one to design the "zodiacal man." The unscientific espousal of astrology prevented the advance of medicine. For if man's fate was determined by the stars, why look any further?

To star-superstition we may now add that of divination. This concept was based upon the theory that everything in nature that shows some form of action has an inborn intelligence and a definite plan. Many objects have been used for divination, but the organs of sacrificed animals were the most preferred. Of these, the liver was most used, particularly that of sheep. An examination of the fresh organ was made. Any deviation from normal in color, shape, size, or form had prognostic value for either being a good or bad omen. While this superstition was as valueless as astrology, it was the beginning of the study of anatomy.

In this world of evil supernatural forces, there was little opportunity for a sensible approach and sane method to practice medicine. "Chaldean wisdom" predominated, a system predicated on religion, astrology, magic, and divination. With such a background, the medical field was filled with magicians, wizards, conjurors, witches, sorcerers, diviners, priests, and exorcisers. Rationality would be delayed for many centuries.

The Babylonians believed that all sickness was due to demons entering the human body by the eating of food, drinking of water, or in the inspired air. Getting well was to get rid of the spirit. On the other hand, epidemics or plagues were due to the anger of the gods who punished men for their sins by sending these calamities.

Babylonian healing was of necessity involved with rituals. The patient's body was sprinkled with holy water and anointed with oil. All substances which had come in contact with the patient were burned. The healer was careful to conform with all ceremonialism. On certain days of the month, it was taboo for the physician to touch the patient. Drugs, when given, had to have that magic touch that could only be imparted if they were collected at specific times and under rigid ritualistic circumstances. The doctor had to be dignifiedly dressed and go through all the formalism of invoking the proper gods such as Ea, Marduk, Ninurta, and Gula to drive out the evil fiend of disease.

In a sense, the assipu was a faith-healer while the asu was a more rational practitioner, but still had to give lip-service to religion and magic. An ancient Babylonian tablet grouped medical practice into three varieties. The first was called *cures* and was essentially in the field of the asu. The second dealt with the masters of the scalpel or knife and referred to surgery, also performed by the asu, although there may have now developed a special branch of physicians called surgeons. The third was exorcism, the exclusive field for the assipu. Prescriptions found on this medical tablet were compounded in conjunction with charms and spells. These liturgies could also be recited before giving the preparation to the patient.

We may assume that the diseases prevailing in the Mesopotamian region today are quite similar to those of three or four thousand years ago. Among these we may mention a few such as smallpox, cholera, typhoid, dysentery, malaria, arthritis, and skin diseases. The usual respiratory disorders, infestations, and cancer were also prevalent, along with a wide variety of infections.

Among medications prescribed by the Babylonians were water, milk, bitters, manna, beer, dates, wine, aloes, cassia, belladonna, castor oil, cinnamon, licorice, mint. mustard, and pomegranate. An eviscerated frog, gall, and curd was applied to the eye for an infection. Because the discharge was yellow, the yellow color of the remedy was thought to be specific. Garlic was widely used for stomach, liver, and intestinal disorders. Oil of cedar was given for scorpion stings, and mallow roots for snake bites. Elaterium was prescribed as a cathartic, sulfur was used for scabies, mustard as a counterirritant, belladonna to relieve pain, dry up saliva, and stop spasm of the intestine, bladder, and uterus. In all, scholars, such as Oefele and Thompson, discovered and identified in the Babylonian tablets over 250 medical plant remedies, over 120 mineral remedies, and over 180 other drugs that were prescribed by the doctors.

Some of the substances used were oils, turpentine, and extracts made from trees such as juniper, cypress, cedar, and laurel. Cactus products were also employed. Resins were derived from myrrh, asafetida, ambra, and galbanum. Vehicles for giving the drugs were water, wine, honey, wax, fat, and milk. Narcotics known in those days were opium, mandrake, and marihuana. Sometimes, sickening nauseating remedies were utilized such as dung of animals, human excrement, and urine. The reason for giving such material was to make demons feel disgusted and leave the body.

Drugs were given as pills, powders, poultices, philters, plasters, and in suppositories. Bandages and splints were known and utilized. Eye medicine was applied from a bronze spatula, and a bronze catheter was used for removing urine when the bladder was distended. The Babylonians knew how to apply massage and cupping. They were also skillful in blood letting, known medically as venesection.

Fire and water were the elements most frequently used in driving out demons. Fire was a sacred substance and a purifier. Antidemonic items were thrown into the fire to help drive away the devils. Of course incantations went along with the procedure. Water was also sacred. After all, it fell from the heavens as a divine offering, and should be used to wash away disease. Strangely, the Babylonian word for water is the word asu. So a physician is one who knows water.

A toothache due to a carious tooth was relieved by packing the cavity with gum mastic and henbane seeds. It was also treated with locally applied mandrake, opium, marihuana, and mustard. Strange to say, the ancients regarded toothache as being caused by a worm which continued to eat away the tooth. This was believed by the Egyptians, Indians, Romans, and Mayans of South America. Modern Arab peasants also hold this opinion.

Babylonians, Hebrews, Egyptians, and the Greeks all considered dreams of much importance. They came from the gods, or in the case of the Hebrews from God. Dreams indicated future happenings. They were omens.

Drugs, Demons, Doctors, and Disease

The Babylonians had developed a great culture. They were astute astronomers and plotted the orbits of the sun, moon, and planets. They knew the equinoxes and solstices. They divided the year into twelve months, the day into twenty-four hours, the minute into sixty seconds. The Babylonians probably invented the water clock and sundial. They were skilled in engineering, war, and agriculture. They were great builders, scientists, and mathematicians.

Our next subject is ancient Egypt. The Babylonians were more astute in their approach to medicine than the Egyptians, for they applied their broad knowledge of mathematics and astronomy to the subject. The Egyptians, on the other hand, depended on folklore and stories handed down from their ancestors to guide them. It is true that both relied on magic and religion and that is what they had in common. Another point of difference is in their prescriptions. Babylonian records were short and mentioned the drug to be used, leaving the quantity to be administered up to the practitioner. The Egyptian records, on papyrus, were long and detailed and gave the exact quantities of the drug to be used.

All knowledge of the ancient Egyptians was contained in the Sacred Books, exactly 42 of them, according to Clement of Alexandria. Legend attributes these books as a gift from the god Thoth. The last six books were on anatomy, drugs, disease, and instruments. They were the complete guides for practicing medicine by the priests in early Egypt. For this was a sacred duty and only the priests were physicians.

Next to Thoth in the healing hierarchy were the gods Serapis and Apis, the so-called inventors of medicine. These gods, like the famous Imhotep, were once living men and had been deified after their death. Imhotep was considered the greatest physician of Egypt and lived around 2980 B.C. He was the patron god, the father of Egyptian medicine.

The priests of Egypt did not improvise when treating patients. They followed the instructions completely as laid down in the Sacred Books. The main forms of therapy consisted of divination and magic.

Our major source of medical knowledge of ancient Egypt comes from various papyri discovered in Egypt during the last century. Most of these texts refer to older texts going back a thousand years or more. The Kahun papyrus is about 4,000 years old and deals with gynecology. The Smith papyrus is about 3700 years old and is a surgical treatise. The Ebers papyrus is about 2500 years old and is concerned with human organs and disease. It prescribes the necessary incantations and charms to be used and closes with a short surgical section.

According to the papyri, the Egyptians attributed disease to supernatural causes and this called for treatment by religious and magic methods. Surgical diseases, were due to natural occurrences such as injury and external trauma. These concepts continued down to our Middle Ages. In the Jewish Talmud there is a similar belief, namely, that some diseases are due to human causes and others sent by a displeased Providence.

Egyptian therapeutics were based upon the belief that the drugs in themselves were not curative. But the remedies had been prepared and used by the gods themselves; therefore, if prepared properly, divine influences would accompany their administration. The rituals accompanying the giving of medicines were the real healing powers. There were magic words, prayers to the gods, and the gods were even threatened with destruction and privations if they did not cooperate with the healer. All these psychologic capers appealed to the patient and he firmly believed the demon would be driven out.

Like the Babylonians, the Egyptians had their healing gods. Thoth, the moon god, was a specialist in eye diseases. He is credited with discovering the enema by seeing an ibis used its beak to inject water into its rectum. Neith was the patroness of physicians. She helped in childbirth, could turn away demons from sleepers, brought disorders by the desert wind. Isis, the earth goddess, was a great healer, even bringing the dead back to life. Seth not only healed but also spread disease. Ptah was concerned with his people's health. Ra, god of the sun, and chief god in the hierarchy, was the discoverer of medicine. The Egyptian gods, unlike the Babylonians, were not immune from disease and suffered like humans. However, they could treat and cure one another. The literature in the temples preserved, for the people, the remedies that the gods used for themselves.

The priests were physicians and so we have a class of healers who possessed the divine knowledge to cope with disease. Medicine was taught in the temples along with other priestly knowledge. The most famous of these "medical schools" were at On, Sais, Thebes, and Memphis. Here priests were taught that a special demon is associated with the disease which attacks a specific part of an individual. These demons, vampires, or ghosts, or even the spirits of the dead, entered the body by natural openings such as the mouth, nose, ears, or rectum. Certain articles, minerals, stones, and plants had healing powers given by the gods and could be used to combat disease.

It might be mentioned that the word "brain" was first expressed in the human language in the Smith Papyrus, although the initial study of the brain was credited to Alkmaeon about 500 B.C. The Egyptian physician, who is unknown, described the anatomy of the brain, knew it was the seat of consciousness, while others in his day and recent times considered the heart the seat of the psyche.

With the passage of time, it became evident that certain drugs seemed to be associated with natural curative powers, lost their superstitious value, and were considered to be natural remedies. Disorders which were more difficult to cure needed the magic treatment. Incantations were utilized. Spells were invoked along with the tying of magic knots or the preparation of healing amulets which would be worn. Especially effective was a knot tied seven times, for seven was a magic number. This knot could be worn around the neck as well as enchanted beads, charms, or other blessed fetishes. All this nonsense had a powerful psychological influence on the patient.

There were three types of healers — physicians, surgeons, and the exorcists. The first used remedies for both internal and external conditions. The surgeons treated fractures, wounds, and dislocations. They were skilled in the use of the knife, cautery, and the suturing of wounds. They knew how to set fractures and apply splints and plaster bandages. When wounds were infected they employed remedies such as extract of willow, solutions of copper and sodium salts, grease, fresh meat, honey, and the dung of various animals.

The third class of healers were the exorcists who worked their healing by magic, amulets, and spells. While demonic spirits were the main antagonists to be fought, there was a beginning of recognition that disease "pests" could be carried to people by the winds, flies, gnats, mosquitoes, geese, asses, and other animals.

In the Ebers papyrus, prescriptions are similar to those of modern times. The physicians gave pills, used extracts of various drugs, and liquids. To dissolve drugs they employed water, milk, beer, and wine. Honey was added, like syrups in modern times, to make the medications sweet and therefore more palatable. Ointments, suppositories, and powders were also known. The Egyptians were fond of enemas and laxatives, for in this way they believed they were keeping their bodies very clean internally. They possessed a number of cathartic preparations, and favorites were senna and castor oil, which they are credited with discovering.

Eye conditions were very prevalent in Egypt, possibly because of the hot deserts and the stinging winds which blew off them. For inflamed eyes they employed malachite, resin, myrrh and burned papyri, possibly the latter had some magic quality. For trachoma, red and yellow ochre and red natron were popular. For leukoma, it was bile. Other preparations utilized were milk, urine, and the blood of a bat or lizard.

Remedies for other conditions were as follows. Roundworms and tapeworms were the common infestors in the country. To combat them, turpentine and pomegranate root were prescribed. Rectal disorders were treated with local applications, enemas, injections, and suppositories. Baldness was treated with a mixture of fats from a lion, hippo, crocodile, goose, serpent and ibex. Another remedy was an equal mixture of ink and spinal fluid. A third formula was a preparation consisting of phallic and vulval tissues mixed with a black lizard. Perhaps this was a last ditch method to cure baldness by using the sexual tissues of both male and female. Bullock's bile and ostrich egg were beaten up in fresh milk and applied to the face for acne.

Disorders of women were treated by having a woman stand over hot coals upon which perfumed wax had been placed. This scented smoke was to lure the womb back to its normal position, for the ancients believed it moved about and thus produced symptoms. According to the number of prescriptions in the papyri, Egyptian women suffered a great deal from gynecologic diseases. The idea of fumigation persisted throughout the ages, even until this century, when girls were advised to get menstrual relief by urinating into a bucket of hot coals and letting the resultant steam fumigate their genitals. Such advice was given by grandmothers early in the nineteen-hundreds. The Egyptians prohibited birth control and abortion. Yet, in the Kahun Papyrus certain contraceptive information is given. One recommendation is the insertion of a vaginal suppository containing honey, crocodile dung, and sodium bicarbonate. The Ebers papyrus recommends tips of gum arabic, which when in contact with the vaginal secretion, produced lactic acid. This acid has been incorporated into modern contraceptive jellies, for it is effective.

Egyptians were a very hygienic people, bathing very frequently and wearing simple linen dress which they changed quite often. They avoided flatulent foods like pork, beans, and onions for they believed these foods upset the intestinal tract, and, to them, excessive food intake was the chief cause of natural illness. Therefore, they took frequent enemas and laxatives to clean out the bowels.

About 700 drugs are mentioned in their texts. They used animal, vegetable, and mineral substances, even human blood, brain, and heart. Among the animals utilized were asses, bats, birds, chickens, ducks, fish, frogs, geese, goats, lions, lizards, mice, snakes, and turtles. Animal excretions such as mucus, saliva, urine, and feces were employed. Even flyspecks were considered therapeutic and given for colic.

Plants and trees were used and no parts were thrown away. Among them were acacia, anise, barley, cassia, cinnamon, dates, figs, garlic, juniper, lotus, onion, peas, poppy (opium), saffron, sunflower, mustard and willow buds.

Water was held in high regard. This was only natural because of the Egyptian concept that the human body was a miniature replica of the universe. The latter was composed of earth, water, fire and wind. In the human the solid elements representing the earth were the flesh and bones. The fluids of the body were like the waters of the Nile. The heat of the body represented fire, and respiration the winds.

Various types of water were recommended and they were identified. In prescriptions, the waters employed were plain water, spring water, well water, bird-pond water, rain water and, ridiculously, the most potent water was that in which the penis was washed. Beer, like water, was regarded as being therapeutic. Among the types utilized were plain beer, bitter beer, flat beer, cold beer, frothy beer, and beer brewed from mixed ingredients. Of course, yeast was good, too. Milk was also a valuable remedy and human milk was considered the best of all.

Minerals known to the Egyptians and used in medicine were alum, arsenic compounds, bicarbonate of soda, salt, limestone, iron oxide, and salt. These substances were applied to the skin for

Drugs, Demons, Doctors, and Disease

various disorders. Soothing materials such as acacia and frankincense were also placed on the skin. Alkaline preparations, along with bland mucilaginous substances, were administered for stomach and ulcer pain.

Eventually, in the long history of ancient Egypt, non-priestly men took up the practice of medicine. Egyptian physicians became very famous and were much sought in antiquity. Even the poet Homer refers to them in his Odyssey composed around 1000 B.C., and Herodotus, the great Greek historian, who lived about 500 B.C., tells us that both Persian kings, Cyrus and Darius, used Egyptian physicians. All Egyptian physicians were specialists in some branch of medicine. Egyptian medicine reached its height around the 18th dynasty, about 1500 B.C. Then it deteriorated into magic and sorcery, but still was highly respected even around 500 B.C. by Herodotus, and the Greeks went to Egypt to study medicine. But decline continued and during the Alexandrian period the situation was reversed, the Egyptians went to Greece to study medicine.

The importance of Egyptian medicine is its contributions to the Greeks. Greek medicine, which we will discuss shortly, got its foundation in Egypt. Homer tells of the skill of the Egyptian physicians in preparing drugs and their chemical knowledge. The word "chemi" refers to the "Black Land," which was the ancient name for Egypt. The science of compounding drugs was known as the Black Art.

The origin of the Hebrews and Abraham is clouded in antiquity. From Sumerian accounts it is known that there were some nomads called Habiru around 2000 B.C. The name Hapiru appears in Egyptian texts, and Habiru in Hurrian texts of Assyria. It is now believed that the earliest Hebrews were related somehow to the widely-spread people known as the Habiru. In the Bible, Eber, great-grandson of Shem, is believed to be the eponymous ancestor of the Hebrews. The name Hebrew also signifies one who has come from the other side of the River, the Euphrates.

Abraham, or Abram as he is also known, came from Ur in the Chaldees and Harran, both cities being centers for moon worship. Called by God, he left his home to settle in Canaan. The early Habiru or Hebrews were affected by the cultures in which they lived, such as the Sumerian, Accadian, Babylonian, Egyptian, and Assyrian. Undoubtedly the early Hebrews were pagans living in pagan lands. Yet, they eventually developed the monotheistic concept of Jehovah or Yahweh.

The early Hebrews believed in the demonic theory of diseases and, being ruled by priests, had no need for physicians. However, physicians came into use later and were, unlike the Egyptian specialists, general practioners. Dreams and magic played a great role in the lives of these people. It was believed that he who did not dream was not in favor with God. Magic is mentioned in the Bible where Moses and Aaron performed miracles in Egypt at the court of Pharoah to free the Israelites.

The Hebrews entertained a supernatural concept regarding medical illness. Sickness, disease, and early death resulted from offending God, and represented punishment for violating some religious law. Epidemics visited a community because of the sins of their leader or the transgressions of the people. Atonement could be made by prayers, sacrifices, and repentance under the leadership of the prophets or priests. The anger of the Lord in the Bible is demonstrated by leprosy being inflicted on Miriam, Uzziah, and Gehazi, the plagues visited on Egypt, the plague cast on the Philistines, the death of Lot's wife, and the death of the first born of David and Bathsheba.

Moses, the great lawgiver and prince of Egypt, brought with him from Egypt the "wisdom of the Egyptians." In Leviticus are recorded his laws of hygiene, conduct, and sex. What foods were permitted and forbidden are mentioned, being based on sound medical knowledge. Jewish medicine before and after the Exodus was Egyptian.

Eventually physicians, not priests, ministered to the people. Yet there is no mention anywhere in the Bible of a famous practicing physician by name. The prophets were versed in folk medicine and often used their knowledge. Elisha and Elijah gave artificial respiration in mouth to mouth resuscitation and this is the first mention of the procedure in any literature.

After the Babylonian captivity, the Jews showed the influence of Babylonian medicine in tneir treatments. During the Hellenic era, Greek influence predominated. Jews studied medicine in Alexandria, the greatest cultural capital in the ancient world. Still, Jewish physicians did not gain fame until the Middle Ages. The priests enforced the hygenic codes and the law, the physicians treated surgical conditions and natural diseases.

Drugs, Demons, Doctors, and Disease

The drugs used by the ancient Hebrews were probably the same as those employed by the Egyptians and Babylonians. The Bible does not mention a pharmacopeia, such as we have found in the writings of these other people. Drugs noted in it, however, are cassia, balm of Gilead, myrrh, sweet spices, storax, mandrake (as an aphrodisiac), nitre, various balsams, laudanum (opium), oil, wine, tragacanth. Wine was used as a depressant. Oil was applied to bruises, infected sores, and wounds. The balms were also used to heal wounds.

Cupping, leeching, and bloodletting were common. A draught, possibly opium or a large amount of wine was given before surgery to deaden the senses. The physicians performed operations such as amputations, Caesarian sections to deliver a live child from a dead mother, removal of the spleen, skull operations, and many others. Women were delivered on a birth stool as in Egypt or on the lap of a midwife or relative. Birth control and abortion were sacriligious.

Fractures and dislocations were treated; artificial limbs, dentures, and crutches were supplied.

The Essenes, a branch of the Pharisees, believed they could call on beneficial spirits to drive out evil demons. Because of their devotion to God, they felt that they could invoke divine power to cure the lame, blind, and the deaf. They utilized prayers, charms, incantations, and magic symbols when a fellow Essene became sick. Drugs and herbs were used only as an aid to spiritual therapy.

In the New Testament, healing is of the miraculous type. No medications are used. Jesus heals by divine power as the Son of God. Luke, alone of the disciples, is a physician, and he records many of these miracles.

The Gospels and Acts demonstrate two different causes for disease. First and foremost is the idea that all disease and sickness is inflicted upon man by God as punishment for sin. Secondly, illness is due to a demon being present in the body.

Healing of the sick is one of the important duties mentioned in the New Testament. James (5:14, 15) states that if one is sick he should call the elders of the church to pray for and anoint him in the name of the Lord. The prayer offered in faith will save the sick individual and the Lord shall raise him up again. If we confess our sins to one another, and pray for one another, then we will be healed. A good man's prayer is powerful and effective.

Drugs, Demons, Doctors, and Disease

In modern medicine there is a place for the physician and a place for the minister.

In ancient times, medicine and surgery were far advanced in India. In fact, India led the world in surgery. Susruta was the ancient world's greatest plastic surgeon, restoring new noses to Indians who had lost theirs as a punishment for crimes.

Two of India's greatest physicians, Susruta and Charaka, mention hundreds of plants with medical uses. They knew that stramonium would relieve asthma, nux vomica was good for dyspepsia, arsenic for intermittent fever, and mercury for syphilis. They prescribed a low salt diet for nephritis (kidney disease), and a high calorie diet for tuberculosis. Wines were employed for surgical anaesthesia. In many respects the ancient Indian pharmacopeia was valueless and contained many disgusting remedies. However it did possess some valuable items. Seaweed was prescribed for goitre, ephedrine for hay fever and asthma, mercury for skin disease and syphilis. Among some of the drugs known and used by Indian physicians were pomegranate, opium, cassia, ginger, acacia, castor oil, croton oil (powerful carthartic), cinnamon, chenopodium (worm killer), marihuana, garlic, honey, sugar, peppers and sesame.

Various parts of plants were utilized such as blossoms, bark, juices, leaves, fruits, twigs, resins and oils. Animal substances made use of were bile, blood, urine, meat (especially fowl and buffalo), sperm, claws, bone, nails, and sinews. Milk was considered most valuable, and human milk was the best.

Chemical drugs employed were antimony, mercury, copper, lead, iron, sulphur, salt, aluminum, potassium, gold, silver, and tin.

For surgical anesthesia, the physicians administered wine, opium, and the burning fumes of hemp (marihuana). Susruta mentions henbane (hyoscyamus) and Indian hemp known as cannabis indica or marihuana. An inhalation anesthetic was described by an Indian physician many centuries later which he called sammohini and which is unknown to us. Certain potions were also prescribed which were given orally and produced deep sleep and abolished all pain during surgery.

Drugs were prepared for use in many forms. Among these were pills, powders, liquids such as syrups, tinctures or alcoholic extracts, lotions, ointments, plasters, suppositories, oils and emulsions, sprays and steam inhalations.

The Indians, Persians, and Chinese knew how to vaccinate against smallpox long before the Western world. They used pus from the smallpox pustule. The Chinese placed the pus upon a piece of cotton and inserted it into the left nostril for boys, and into the right nostril for girls. Why the discrepancy we do not know.

According to anthropologists, Indian civilization is one of the oldest on earth. About three or four thousand years B.C., there was evidence of a high grade culture in India, about the equal of the Sumerians. The Aryans invaded India in 1600 B.C. and in the process became civilized. The oldest known period of Indian medicine dates from 1600 to 800 B.C. and is called the Vedic period. Indian beliefs repeat the same story again, namely, that disease is supernatural in origin. Demons cause disease, and even the healing gods may do likewise. Physicians were known during this period and were divided into surgeons, regular physicians, magicians, and sorcerers.

The second period of Indian medicine is known as the Brahman. During this interval, extending to around 1000 A.D., Hindu medicine reached its highest peak. The three greatest physicians were Charaka, Susruta, and Vaghbata. As to the exact time in which they lived, no unanimity of opinion exists. Some claim that Charaka lived around 1000 B.C. and Susruta anywhere from 600 B.C. to 600 A.D. One of the greatest medical works is ascribed to Susruta and is known as the Susruta Samhita. In addition to surgery, it gives treatment for medical conditions.

According to Susruta, the human body consists of humors, excretions, and fundamental principles. Translated by Western physicians these are identified as air, bile and phlegm. Let us remember this when we get to Graeco-Roman medicine. Susruta describes many well known diseases. Illness is due to disturbances of the three humors (air, bile, and phlegm). Philosophy, religion, medicine, mythology, magic, incantations, charms, are all blended together in this great work, the Samhita.

Charaka's book, the Charaka Samhita, is primarily a medical text Many medicines are described in it. The importance of dreams is stressed. Diet, seasons, and living habits influence the development and course of a disease by exciting the basic humors of air, bile and phlegm.

Vagbata's main work is the Astranga Samgraha. It is quite similar to the previous works, especially Susruta's. Vagbata lived probably about 700 A.D.

Drugs, Demons, Doctors, and Disease

In surgery, the ancient Hindus exceeded all others. Their plastic surgery of the face was outstanding, notably that of the nose, ears and lips. They used hair as sutures. They knew how to remove metal iron splinters with a magnet. They performed good abdominal surgery, using ants as sutures by allowing them to bite into the intestines to close wounds and then their heads were snipped off.

The Indians knew how to use hypnosis. Patients were often taken to the temples to be treated by this method. Hypnotism was introduced by the English into Europe in the last century, being imported from India.

The first known hospitals were Indian, being in existence about 500 B.C. King Ashoka, in the third century B.C., erected two kinds of hospitals, one for men and one for animals. His deeds were carved on rocks, and on them are also recorded the numerals which centuries later were called Arabic, but which the Arabs did not invent.

The third period of Indian medicine is Mongol, for these savage invaders came into India in the seventh century of our era. Their rule continued until the British conquest. Moslem physicians practiced along with Hindus. Under Moslem rule Indian medicine declined.

Surgery was well practiced in ancient India. The surgeons knew how to remove tonsils, cataracts, and limbs. Operations for removal of bladder stones were performed as well as hemorrhoidectomies (excision of piles). Suturing material was made from flax, hemp, hair and also bark fibers. Straight and curved needles were employed. The physicians had good knowledge of the techniques of cupping, leeching, cauterization, and blood letting. There is evidence that they knew something of nerve surgery and even went into the skull to explore for disorders. They possessed a vast array of surgical instruments.

There is evidence of medical schools being set up in the country to train physicians and surgeons. They were located at Benares and Taxil.

Like the Hebrews and Egyptians, the Hindus practiced scrupulous hygiene. Their rules prescribed frequent bathing, diet, exercise, and internal cleanliness by emetics, laxatives, and an occasional venesection or bloodletting. After each meal, toothpicks were used to clean the teeth and the mouth rinsed with medications or solutions made from herbs.

Because ancient Hindu and Greek medicine were contemporary, the question was often raised as to which borrowed from which. There is evidence in antiquity that there was commercial trading between the Indians and the Egyptians, Babylonians, and the Hebrew King Solomon. It is quite logical to assume that the Greeks also traveled to India. In the fourth century B.C. Alexander the Great invaded India. While the question may never be completely solved, we will see contemporary knowledge among the Greeks.

The beginning of Greek medicine is lost in antiquity. Initially, it must have been Stone Age medicine. Possibly, it derived some benefits from the Minoan and Mycenaean civilizations which preceded it. Probably, Egyptian and Babylonian borrowings gave the Greeks the impetus they needed. Whether Indian medicine contributed anything is still speculative. If we had to choose what most scholars feel is the main source of Grecian medical knowledge, we would say it was Egyptian. The Greek gods, Apollo, Athena, Hermes, and Aesculapius are definitely related to their Egyptian counterparts.

The initial period of ancient Greek medicine is known as Aesculapian medicine. Aesculapius is the Greek Imhotep, a physician who became a god. After being deified, the myth arose that Aesculapius was the son of Apollo and a beautiful, mortal girl named Coronis. So skillful in medicine and surgery was he, that he not only cured the sick and wounded, but healed the dying and brought back life to the dead. Zeus, king of the gods, feared that man would now become immortal and so he slew Aesculapius with one of his thunderbolts. Regretting his action, Zeus raised Aesculapius to godhood.

For hundreds of years, people flocked to the temples of Aesculapius to be healed. While asleep, in the temple, the god would supposedly visit them in a dream and advise them how they could be cured. It is not known whether the induced sleep was produced by hemlock or the poppy seed (opium). This system of healing was based primarily upon miracles, hypnosis, and suggestion. In addition to this treatment, the patients received special baths, fasting diets, and laxatives, but these preceded the temple sleep and were purifications. The most famous temple of Aesculapian healing was at Epidaurus. The temple grounds contained a theatre seating 20,000 people, a stadium for 12,000 spectators, and shrines to Aesculapius

Drugs, Demons, Doctors, and Disease

and his daughter, Hygeia. Mineral baths were available, also a hostel and library.

Before being admitted for treatment, the patient was completely examined. If he appeared too sick, he was not accepted. If an admitted patient grew seriously ill and might die, he was carried out of the temple into the woods and left to die. For it was claimed by the priests that nobody ever died in the temple, and they did not want their god to appear anything but infallible. Fees were charged, and the people were only too glad to freely give in order to be cured. The skill of Aesculapius was due to a sacred snake, which gave him a magic herb to cure all sickness. Snakes were prevalent around the grounds of the temple, and, during the temple-sleep, the god frequently appeared as a snake. Snakes have always fascinated man and supposedly possessed some mystical qualities. As a result, the symbol of Aesculapius became two snakes intertwined on a staff and known as the caduceus, which is the modern medical symbol derived from the Greeks.

Gods, as in other cultures, had power over disease, health, and life itself. In tribal days, local gods were appealed to for help when sickness arose. Later, certain gods were identified with the healing arts. Zeus sent disease, very seldom provided healing. His daughter Athena was not clearly defined in healing. Apollo was originally a sender or restrainer of plagues, later a healer. His sister Artemis was the women's healer as well as the cause of their nervous and psychologic disorders. Dionysus cured by touching. Demeter was outstanding in nursing and in predicting the course of disease. Paieon concerned himself with surgery. Pan's interest was in hygiene and prevention of disease and he could halt a plague. Aesculapius had two daughters, Panacea and Hygeia. The former was capable of healing all diseases with herbs given her by her father. Hygeia was the goddess of hygiene, the guardian of health but not a healer. She was worshipped by the participants in both local athletic games and the Olympic games. According to Homer, Aesculapius had two sons, Machaon and Podalirius, who served as surgeons with the Greek army at Troy.

During the Homeric period of Greek medicine, which existed about 1000 B.C., a great deal of knowledge had been gained from treating battle wounds. Soothing, healing, and pain-relieving drugs were applied to wounds. Skillful surgeons were highly regarded by the contestants. However, internal diseases, where the cause was not obvious, were regarded as being due to evil spirits or the anger of gods and therefore needed supernatural methods to cure. For five or six hundred years after the Trojan war, until the appearance of the Ionian school of philosophers, medicine was mostly controlled by the priests, each devoted to his own healing god. As a result, there was a natural rivalry among them, and this was healthy in advancing medicine, for they had to utilize every available means to accomplish cures, even though their gods were the ones that received credit for the accomplishments.

The philosopher-physicians, most of whom came from the Greek colonies of Ionia in Asia Minor, explored not only medicine but also the universe. They were scientists, or what were formerly called natural philosophers. They were interested in explaining the universe in terms of natural causes and not in anthropomorphic or man-created, theological concepts.

The year 670 B.C. marks the rise of rational medicine in Greece. Psammetichus, the Egyptian Pharoah, allowed Greeks, for the first time, to enter his country and attend Egyptian schools where they learned Egyptian medicine, culture, and science. This favor was granted in return for Greek aid in fighting a civil war. Returning to Greece, these scholars brought back a broad cultural base upon which the agile Greek mind could build.

The Ionian philosophers devised various theories to explain life and matter. Thales of Miletus (650-580 B.C.) believed that all matter was created from water and that the earth floated on water. His pupil, Anaximander, said he was all wrong and that matter was formed from an indestructible prime element, and, furthermore, the earth floated in space. Anaximenes (611-564 B.C.) claimed the prime element was air, for air was life giving. Diogenes of Apollonia (c. 450 B.C.) stated that air was distributed all over the body by the arteries from the heart and aorta. Heraclitus of Ephesus (540-475 B.C.) scoffed at this theory and said that ethereal fire was the chief element of life. He also developed a theory similar to Darwin's on the survival of the fittest. Anaximander devised a Darwinian "origin of the species" idea that life originated in the seas and that man descended from fish which migrated out on land.

These Ionian philosophers tried to explain the universe in terms of matter, motion, and perception. They looked for a basic element. The Eleatics and Pythagoreans were abstractionists and explained the universe in metaphysical terms. Xenophanes, founder of the Eleatics, was a monotheist and attacked the polytheism of the Greeks. He believed that all natural existence could be explained by combinations of the four elements such as water, earth, fire, and air. If these were the components of the entire universe, he reasoned, how were they held together as building blocks? How could particles move in a packed space or vacuum? Did the properties of matter ever change? Was the earth always earth and nothing more, and is this also true of water? Xenophanes was the first person to advance the anatomy of the brain by dissecting various animals. He also believed that the sun and moon were not living things but burning stones.

Democritus (460-350 B.C.) attempted to explain the universe in terms of atoms and space. Atoms he said were indestructible, homogeneous, and in perpetual motion. Even the human body is composed of atoms separated by pores. The atoms circulate in the body, especially in the intestines where they are most active and thereby maintain health. If their circulation is sluggish, or the pores become clogged, or tissues relax due to a decrease in the amount of atoms, then disease results.

Pythagoras was the first Ionian philosopher to write on medical matters. He also said that the earth was a globe revolving from west to east like the planets. He taught that life was made up of four elements—air, fire, earth, and water. Each of these elements possessed a quality such as cold, hot, dry, or moist. These four elements and their four qualities formed the body's four humors. Blood was hot and moist, phlegm was cold and moist. Yellow bile was hot and dry, black bile cold and dry. The relative proportion of these humors determined one's health, disposition, and mental outlook. This humoral theory dominated medical thinking until the middle of the nineteenth century. The terms still linger on as bilious, choleric, phlegmatic, sanguine, or melancholy, the latter meaning black bile.

Pythagoras used medicines to treat the body and music to treat the soul, diseases of the mind, and disorders which occurred in the spring. His pupil, Empedocles, founded the Italian school of medicine, discovered the ear labyrinth, and believed the heart was the center of consciousness in opposition to the idea of Alkmaeon who felt it was in the brain. Empedocles also had an idea that evolution was a mechanical process and that in it, somehow, there was a survival of the fittest.

Euryphon of the school of Cnidus attributed the cause of all disease to improper evacuation of the gastrointestinal tract. Keep the intestines open, he advised, and health would ensue. Euryphon was one of the few doctors of his time who knew that the arteries contained blood, most believing they held air. He taught that hemorrhage came from arteries as well as veins.

While there are many other philosophers and physicians we could discuss, it is fitting now to consider the greatest physician of the Greeks, namely Hippocrates (460-361 B.C.), also known as the father of medicine. He was so honored because he based the science of medicine on personal investigation and clinical experience rather than on superstition, philosophic speculation, and magic. Hippocrates sought the cause of disease in the earthly environment of man, in natural reasons, just like the Ionian philosophers sought to explain the universe and man in natural terms.

Hippocrates carefully examined his patients, recorded their histories and symptoms, and some of his cases are still extant today. He compiled facts and systematized them. He recorded his failures as well as his successes. In studying diseases, he became acquainted with their natural courses and thereby learned to predict which patients would get well and which would die. He said that "Nature heals; the physician is only Nature's assistant". He also felt that he could not tell for sure which drugs had healing properties, and he believed that other doctors exercised their imaginations in deciding which medications to use. Hippocrates, instead of using drugs, sought clean surroundings, good air, and sufficient light for his patients. Diet, baths, and exercise were prescribed as he thought they were needed.

If these measures did not work, he employed purging and emetics such as white hellebore. If still unsuccessful, he resorted to blood letting by cutting into a vein (phlebotomy). The purpose was to prevent and to recall blood when it had taken a supposedly wrong course in the body. Hippocrates used this bleeding technique in dropsy (swelling) due to heart failure and in an attempt to reduce an enlarged spleen. If bleeding and purging both failed, then he tried to induce copious sweating with diaphoretics. Fumigations were ordered for female disorders. Gargles were prescribed for tonsillitis. Other medications used to treat patients were oils, ointments, poultices (cataplasms) and eye medications (collyria).

Hippocrates accepted the humoral theory of Pythagoras and Empedocles, that the body was composed of four primary fluids — blood, yellow bile, black bile, and phlegm. When these were out of adjustment, then disease occurred. His disciples held on to this theory and the great Galen, four hundred years later, strongly endorsed this thinking, which physicians accepted as dogma until late in the last century.

During the time of Hippocrates, there was an intense rivalry between the older medical school at Cnidus in Asia Minor and the new Hippocratic school at Cos, an island in the Aegean Sea and the birthplace of Hippocrates. The older school followed the Egyptian and Babylonian schools, using the drugs and remedies advocated by their predecessors. They also performed surgery in a similar manner. In contrast to the Hippocratic school, they were more concerned with subjective symptoms rather than objective symptoms. While Hippocrates used very few drugs, his surgical treatments were quite advanced. The Cos school of Hippocrates was well ahead in diagnosis, prognosis (predicting the course of disease), surgery, and treatment. They were the world's medical masters and teachers for twenty-three centuries and it is only in the last two hundred years that we have moved ahead of these phenomenal people.

There were other important Greek physicians and philosophers. Some of them were quite ingenious. However, we can not discuss them all. Hippocrates lived during the Golden Age of Greece, the Age of Pericles, which terminated in 404 B.C. when Sparta defeated and ended the rule of sophisticated Athens. The Spartan Empire fell to Thebes in 371 B.C. and, in turn, Thebes and all Greece fell to Alexander the Great, thus initiating the sophisticated and cultural Alexandrian era. Two outstanding physicians, Herophilos and Erasistratos, lived during these times. Herophilos (c. 300 B.C.) was the father of anatomy and dissected many human bodies. After a short while human dissection was forbidden. and not repeated for a thousand years. The other physician, Erasistratos, a younger contemporary of Herophilos, founded the study of physiology based upon anatomy. According to Celsus, both these men dissected live criminals, others doubt these stories. With the death of Cleopatra, the last Ptolemy to rule Egypt was gone, and the Roman Empire eclipsed the Alexandrian Empire.

Roman medicine was inferior to the Greek, and the most desired physicians of the Roman Empire were usually Greek physicians. The native medical theory of the Romans was animistic, completely devoid of any scientific basis. It was a type of folk medicine derived from the aboriginal inhabitants of prehistoric Italy and whatever else was gleaned from the Etruscans, whose civilization preceded the Romans.

Folk healing was widely practiced by priests, sorcerers, elders, old women, weirdos, and people with physical deformities. Roman medicine remained dormant in its pool of superstition and primitivity while Greek medicine was freeing itself from these shackles. For 600 years, the Romans had no physicians. All they had were superstitions which they freely borrowed from other peoples and, as a result, they accumulated a huge inventory of healing gods which governed all diseases. Each ailment had its own god. For example, the god Mars ruled over plagues. Febris was the goddess of malarial fevers. Carna controlled the intestine. The sexual life of women from courtship to pregnancy and nursing was divided among 18 different deities. The Romans finally adopted and took for their own the Greek God Aesculapius. At the time, they were suffering from a pestilence which proved resistant to all their efforts. In desperation, they turned to Aesculapius for help and then the pestilence died out. In gratitude, the Romans built a temple to his honor in Rome and later erected others throughout the empire.

After the Romans conquered the Grecian city of Corinth in 146 B.C., they brought back to Rome many captives among which were some doctors. These and other immigrant Greek physicians soon dominated the medical practice at Rome. Pliny, the Roman writer, defended the dignity of the Romans which did not permit them to practice medicine. He bitterly protested against Romans taking orders from foreign physicians, especially those coming from conquered realms. Anger was expressed by many other Romans at these foreign "medici" as they were called. The first Greek physician finally accepted and honored by the Romans was Asclepiades and, needless to say, Pliny and Galen both hated him.

Medicine in the Roman Republic and during the Imperial period was chiefly Grecian. All medicine worthy of being designated by this term was Grecian from Hippocrates to modern times. Roman medicine was originally practiced by slaves and freedmen, along with barbers and bleeders (phlebotomists). Slaves were instructed in the healing arts and their fees went to their owners. Cato, the Roman statesman, hated all Greek physicians and stated there was no need for doctors anyway. He had his own pet cure-all which will attune itself to some modern ears. It was cabbage. He prescribed it raw, cooked, or as a poultice. He even injected its juice into sinuses and fistulas. Endowed with such supreme ignorance he held all Greek physicians in contempt. Unfortunately, today we still have some modern Catos.

The first Latin medical author was Celsus and he wrote in Latin so that Romans could read his works and not the Greeks. The second author was Scribonius Largus, physician to Emperor Claudius. He followed the methods of Herophilos, using drugs contrary to the practice of the famous Greek physician Asclepiades.

As Hippocrates was considered the father of medicine, so Pedanius Dioscorides (40-90 A.D.) may be thought of as the father of materia medica. He freed drug usage and knowledge from superstition. He utilized scientific investigation in studying vegetable, mineral, and animal substances that were administered to patients. Dioscorides was a Greek from Cilicia and a most famous army surgeon. Due to his extensive travels with Nero's Roman army, he had the opportunity to study the plants of various regions and develop an extensive knowledge of botany.

Dioscorides wrote a book called *De Universa Medicine* in which he gave the properties and actions of over 600 plants, and of these only about 150 were known in the days of Hippocrates. He gave a detailed explanation of each plant, where it came from, what it looked like, and what it was good for in therapy. These plants can be still recognized from the accurate descriptions given by Dioscorides. Until a few years ago, about one hundred of his remedies were still mentioned in the pharmacopeia. For a thousand year after this remarkable man lived, there was practically no progress made in materia medica.

Dioscorides classified his remedies according to their therapeutic effects such as laxatives, digestive agents, diuretics (eliminate water from the body), and sweat producers (diaphoretics). He was the first physician to describe scientifically the opium preparations. He noted their ability to relieve pain, to cause sleep, to quiet coughs, and, in overdoses, to produce lethargy, coma and death. He was the first physician to mention aconite, ammoniacum, and the laxative effects of aloes. He knew that iron had astringent properties and aspidium would be effective against tapeworms.

Dioscorides described many drugs used in the practice of medicine until recently, and some that are still with us. Among these are acacia, alum, ammonia, starch, vinegar, nutgall, silver, marihuana, croton oil, gentian, hyoscamus, mercury, opium, mandragora, salt, peppermint, thyme, tragacanth. He knew of the sleep producing effect of mandragora, hyoscyamus, and opium. He noted the anaesthetic effect of wine of mandragora and its ability to relieve pain. He also suggested that mandragora be given by enema, and stated that in powdered form it can be used locally for anaesthesia. Dioscorides gave detailed instructions for detecting adulteration of drugs. He also recommended certain drugs for birth control and others to cure sterility.

It is most remarkable that the Western Roman Empire produced no great Latin physician. During the Roman Republican era, medical training was available only through being taught by a private physician, and the first important teacher was the Greek physician Aesclepiades, who started a medical school. At first, his school was small and composed of his apprentices and students who followed him about on his visits, and then later he founded a larger school. Soon other schools were created by competitive practitioners. Then the schools merged to form societies or colleges.

Toward the end of Emperor Augustus' reign, these societies built a place for themselves in Rome called the "Schola Medicorum," or school of physicians. It had a president called the "archiatrus" and a secretary known as the "tabularius" or "scriba." Eventually, the emperors built teaching halls or "auditoria." The professors received, as compensation, only the students' fees. Later, in emperor Vespasian's time, (70-79 A.D.) a salary was given. This system was extended by succeeding emperors. The main duties of the archiatrus were to render medical attention to the poor and instruct the students.

Along with free bread and circuses, the Romans experimented with socialized medicine. They had state, circuit, city, and school physicians. The poor had free medical care. The great physician Galen, whom we will discuss shortly, complained that many wealthy

Drugs, Demons, Doctors, and Disease

Roman citizens faked poverty in order to get free medical attention, a practice even carried on in our times.

The practice of medicine was open to anyone. However, those who aspired to high positions such as the archiatrus, chose good courses of study. In time, qualified schools with good teachers opened in various parts of the empire. Among these were the schools at Beneventum and Avranches which, quite remarkably, lasted until the beginnings of the Middle Ages. The best schools became legally recognized and this gradually raised the status of the medical profession. The practice of medicine finally became legalized and a license was necessary to treat patients. Criminal acts such as abortion were punished by loss of one's license and fines.

The Romans had many skilled surgeons and possessed a fine armamentarium of surgical instruments, many of which have been found at Pompeii and other sources. They used lancets, catheters, sounds, vaginal and rectal speculums, forceps, spatulas, scalpels, syringes, rasps, hammers, chisels, probes and other assorted equipment. In the ruins of Pompeii, physicians' offices and surgeries have been excavated. One of these was built along the lines of modern day nursing homes.

The great contribution of Rome to medicine was the development of the hospital system. This arose because of the Roman military establishment being scattered throughout the empire. It was impossible to send soldiers home and so hospitals were built at important sites and medical care rendered there. One such hospital was found at Carnutum, near Vienna. The best preserved is at Novaesium near Dusseldorf in Germany.

The last of the great Roman physicians was Galen, a Greek born in 130 A.D. in Pergamon, a city in Asia Minor. He studied in many medical schools including the world's best at Alexandria. His first appointment was as surgeon to the gladiators at Pergamon, and as a result, he learned much traumatic surgery. He conducted many anatomical and physiological investigations. He proved that the brain was the center of thought and will power. He went to Rome and became the Emperor Marcus Aurelius' personal physician. No other physician has exerted such influence on physicians for 14 centuries as Galen. His word was accepted as gospel truth. He wrote many works on many subjects besides medicine. In the medical field, 85 of his works remain, 45 have been lost. He accepted the four humors theory of Hippocrates and gave them such polish and authority that they survived for fourteen hundred years. Galen's anatomy books were based upon his studies of animal bodies, not humans, and therein lay many reasons for error. But his studies of the skeleton were based upon human observations.

In the use of drugs and knowledge thereof, Galen was not the peer of Dioscorides. Galen, contrastingly, incorporated many drugs in one prescription. He bought formulas from practitioners and other sources and even, strangely, believed in the power of charms and amulets. In contrast to Dioscorides who classified drugs by their actions, Galen classified them by their qualities such as wetness or dryness, heat or cold. Galen was an ordinary surgeon, but his teaching on fractures and dislocations was better than Hippocrates. He described an operation for plastic repair of defects of the lips, nose, and ears.

Galen disclosed a number of novel facts. He told how one could obtain the scent of flowers and plants by distillation. He noted that starlings got fat from eating hemlock, while the same substance was poisonous to man. He observed that poisons from animals such as the asp, viper, or the mucus of a mad dog will not injure a person unless he has an open wound on the skin. He states that Cleopatra knew this and bit her arm first before applying the poison of the asp. The writings of Galen spread throughout the Near East into Persia and the Arab world, being translated into Arabic in the 9th century, and used for about 7 centuries by Hebrew and Arabic scholars. With the exception of adding some new drugs, the physicians living in the Arab countries under Moslem domination did little to advance medicine. Those who stood highest in the history of Arabian medicine were not Arabic but Jews, Persians, Syrians, or Spaniards living under Moslem domination.

The Moslems had been in contact with the Far East since 628 A.D. when they sent a mission to China. Intercourse with China provided them with the Chinese knowledge of healing, chemistry, and the esoteric. As a result, the Arabs became quite proficient in chemistry and pharmacology. Many of our scientific terms are Arabic such as alkali, aldehyde, alchemy, syrups, juleps, and alcohol. Because of their widespread military conquests, as well as their peaceful missions to other lands, the Arabs soon absorbed all the knowledge available on Greek medicine and the drugs of Persia, India, and China. This newly acquired information resulted in the Arabs introducing new medications such as camphor, senna, sandalwood, cloves, cubebs, and ambergris.

With the fall of Rome, Islam acted as the preserver of Greek medicine. Rhazes and Avicenna, both Persians, and the greatest Arabic physicians, added to the Greek heritage with their excellent descriptions of various diseases. Islam, however, by its religious edicts forbade human dissection, autopsy, and vivisection. This prevented any advancement of anatomy and physiology, and consequently there could be no medical progress. In the sciences, where no such restrictions existed, the Arabic world contributed to the advancement of mathematics, architecture, and astronomy. After the fall of the Western Roman Empire, a cultural and educational darkness fell on the European continent until the Renaissance. Arabic became the scientific language of men and was to the world of that time what Greek had been in the previous thousand years.

We have one other culture to mention before we move up to modern times, and that is Chinese. For millenia, China isolated herself from all nations. Also, there was a racial barrier between her and the Western cultures. In a sense, she was and is a loner, and unique in her philosophical concepts. The Chinese philosophers believed in a dual control of nature, the yang and the yin. The yang represented the male, active, positive, perfect essence of heaven, the sun, day, and heat principle. The yin was the female, inactive, passive, imperfect essence, moon, earth, night and cold principle. The interplay of these forces was responsible for all activities in heaven, earth, religion, crafts, and medicine. The same was true for living and non-living things.

Animate and inanimate substances were made up of five prime elements, in addition to the yang and yin principles. These were fire, wood, metal, earth, and water. During the process of creation, they were all derived from water. Man was considered by the philosophers to be a miniature replica of the universe, a microcosm of heaven and earth, which represented a blending of animal and spiritual souls. The animal portion of the soul was the lower, coarser, cruder component. The spiritual portion was the higher, softer, erudite part. Man was created by the vital essence in which both the yang and yin merged in proper proportions. This concept was also applied to foods, herbs, and drugs. The life-invigorating and healing substances had more yang than yin, while those possessing the reverse were disease-producing, unhealthy substances.

Because of this philosophic thinking, the Chinese regarded health as a proper equilibrim between yang and yin as well as a proper coordination between the five prime elements. The male principle was warm and dry, and the female principle was cold and moist. The male principle held control over the stomach, intestines, and bladder, the female resided in the solid organs such as the liver, kidneys, lungs, heart, and spleen. When one died his dual soul dispersed, the yang to heaven, the yin to the earth. Thus the souls of all departed lived both in heaven and on earth. As a result, the Chinese paid great respect to their ancestral dead. This devotion prevented any dissection of the honored dead, and, together with the yang and yin philosophy, there was no reason to do any research or delve into the physiology or pathology of disease. It was already explained.

The Chinese did not create medical schools for training doctors. Medicine was a hand-me-down from father to son. Therefore, everything that was old was good and everything that was new was bad. The Chinese materia medica, known as the Pen Ts'ao, goes back to prehistoric times. Chinese therapeutics were based on the thinking that in nature there existed a remedy for every disorder. The substance was effective as long as it was not antagonistic to religious faith. Consequently, every possible substance was tried and used whether it was animal, vegetable, or mineral. Drugs were used for internal treatments, external therapy consisted of acupuncture and moxa. Religious treatment involved the wearing of amulets, paying homage to pictures of the gods, and prayers to the divinities and demons.

Acupuncture and Moxibustion were Chinese inventions. There were over 350 points on the body which the experienced Chinese acupuncture physician could puncture with needles, either hot or cold, to treat certain disorders. The purpose was to unlock stagnant points in the body, allow the harmful humors to leave the body, and permit fresh beneficial humors to get in. This procedure was very ancient. In a sense, it might be considered similar to counter-irritation by the use of liniments, hot poultices, and hot applications. Moxibustion may be considered more so. Moxa was made by rolling leaves of mugworth into small balls. They were placed upon properly designated spots on the skin and then lighted. When they

Drugs, Demons, Doctors, and Disease

burned the skin, the glowing masses were forced into the blisters which had resulted from the burns. Sometimes acupuncture was followed by moxibustion.

Among the most esteemed drugs used in Old China, the ginseng root held the highest virtue. It was considered a vital plant which could extend one's years. Another plant with so-called similar properties is the shang-luh. Other popular drugs were pomegranate for worms; rhubarb and camphor for constipation; iron, aconite, and marihuana for anemia; copper and betonia for emesis; sulfur for skin aliments; croton, pigs gallbladder, plums for laxatives; aloes, snake skins, bat dung, and rhubarb for dysentery; tiger testicles and stag horn marrow for sexual impotency; cinnamon, opium, ginger for bronchial disorders; red lead and powdered horns of antelope for heart trouble; dragon bones, hair, and ginger for hemorrhage.

The Chinese used animal organs to treat the identical diseased human organs. Predominate among these were the lungs, kidneys, spleen, and liver. Animal excreta and secretions, rather a repulsive and odious therapy, were given for various disorders, in the manner of the ancient Egyptians. The Chinese feared demons and used drugs, amulets, and prayers to ward them off. Sorcerers used shang-luh to fight off and even slay demons.

The Chinese made some discoveries which are admirable, although most of their materia medica was useless. They used seaweed, with its iodide content, to treat goitre. Ephedrine was given for hay fever for over 5,000 years and is now used in the West for asthma. They used mercury ointments for skin diseases. The Chinese claimed to be the first to use smallpox pus for inoculation against the disease itself. Pig liver with its high content of vitamin A was administered for night blindness.

Chinese medicine because of its insularity and religious restrictions was bound to stagnate. However this ancient system is still widely practiced in China today, being favored over western medicine by the die-hard revolutionaries. Chinese surgery, restricted in the same manner as medicine, also retrogressed. While the Chinese considered all disease due to the altered relationship between the yang and yin, they did consider contributing causes such as atmospheric changes, religious and demonic influences, over-indulgence in eating, drinking, and sex, taking of poisonous substances, and emotional disturbances such as anger, jealousy, and passion.

Chapter Three

MEDIEVAL MEDICINE

THE MIDDLE AGES MAY BE considered as that period between the fall of Rome and the beginning of the rebirth of the intellect, known as the Renaissance. This is approximately the interval between the fifth and fifteenth centuries.

While the medieval period was one in which great cathedrals were built, famous universities were founded, and the Church was supreme, it was a sterile period for medicine and the famous medical historian Singer called it a time of "progressive deterioration of the intellect". Sarton, however, objects and names prominent physicians during this period such as Avicenna and Rhazes. Nevertheless, the climate was definitely not one to stimulate intellectualism at a time when ignorance was rampant both in the educational and ecclesiastical realms, whether they were Christian, Jewish, or Moslem and the penalty for transgression was death.

The Arabic world became finally divided into the Eastern and Western Caliphates. In the Eastern Caliphate, the outstanding physician was Rhazes (841-926) who wrote the first articles on smallpox, measles, and hay fever. He was followed by Haley Abbas who described common skin diseases and their treatments. Next followed Avicenna (980-1037) known as the Leonardo da Vinci of the Arab world. He was a most remarkable man. He is said to have been the first one to describe the properties of alcohol and sulfuric acid. He stated that wine was the best dressing for wounds. He left an excellent description of diabetes and noted the sweetishness of diabetic urine. His most famous work is his medical text called the *Canon* which gave detailed and vivid descriptions of many medical diseases. It was used for over 500 years in the West as the standard textbook in medical schools. Avicenna attacked astrology as being useless, even while it was firmly being embraced by Western physicians.

In the Western Caliphate, the greatest physician was Avenzoar of Cordova (1091-1162) who was considered the Avicenna of the East. He discredited Galenism. He was among the first parasitologists to describe the itch mite of scabies, previously mentioned by Alexander of Tralles (526-605), who was the first to recommend rhubarb for intestinal worms and colchicum for gout, a remedy used even today. Avenzoar was followed by his pupil Averroes (1126-1198) who built a system of medicine based upon Aristotle's philosophy. His most famous pupil was Maimonides (1135-1208), a famous philosopher and physician, who became physician to Saladin and wrote a book for his son on dieting and personal hygiene. Maimonides' books on aphorisms, poisons, asthma, and hemorrhoids were translated from Arabic and widely circulated throughout Europe. The Western Caliphate finally fell to the Christians who absorbed the Islamic culture. The Eastern Caliphate unfortunately fell to the savage murdering Mongols who destroyed everything in their path and obliterated all learning.

With the founding of a medical school at Salerno, Italy, in 1072, medicine began its slow upward climb in Europe, to finally rise from the depths of ignorance, superstition, and ineptitude. This school blended four influences, namely, Greek, Latin, Hebrew, and Islamic. The Arabic authority lasted until the seventeenth century. The success of the school inspired the founding of new schools, at Paris (1110), Oxford (1167), Bologna (1158), Padua (1222), and other cities.

During the Middle Ages, the people of Europe were stricken with very severe epidemics. The great and little minds of those days attributed these violent outbreaks to stars, comets, droughts, freezes, storms, crop failures, floods, insects, poisoning of wells by Jews, and other absurdities. The real factors were the miserable crowding of the people along with the horrible sanitation of the walled towns. These conditions aided and abetted the spread of disease organisms. The filth, squalor, and uncleanliness of the masses, and their intermingling in common bath houses, helped to disperse infections. Europe was also teaming with wandering soldiers, vagabonds, students, peddlers, and other ramblers who moved from town to town disseminating their infectious germs.

Among the great epidemics which swept over Europe were leprosy, St. Anthony's fire (ergotism), sweating sickness (influenza), St. Vitus dance (epidemic chorea), syphilis, and the Black Death (bubonic plague). Leprosy and influenza were believed to have been spread or introduced by the Crusaders. In fact, influenza was considered to be due to cosmic "influence" (influentia coeli) and this is how it got its name. St. Anthony's fire was often mistakenly diagnosed as being due to ergot ingestion, when it was actually erysipelas. Frequently, there was confusion between the bubonic plague and other diseases. Psoriasis was misdiagnosed leprosy. The Black Death first spread over Asia, then moved into Europe about 1348. Before it quieted down, it killed over 60 million people. It again broke out sporadically, but never reached such decimating proportions.

Syphilis was the next great epidemic. It was supposed to have first occurred at the siege of Naples in 1495 and given to the French by Columbus' sailors who were assumed to have brought it from the New World. Karl Sudhoff, famous medical historian, states that this story is untrue and that syphilis was known in Europe before Columbus. The disease was not recognized as a distinct entity at first. Later, its venereal transmission was recognized. Mercury was used to treat the condition. Various reasons were assigned for the disease such as astrological phenomena, rains, intercourse of a leper with a prostitute, and the poisoning of wells. Because of the vast outbreak of the disease, it soon became clear that it was being spread by sexual intercourse. Yet syphilis continued to flourish, racing along with tuberculosis and alcoholism in gathering in its victims.

Medical practice during the Renaissance was bound up with superstition, herb-doctoring, and of course quackery. The theological concepts of disease indicated a devil for each disease and a special saint to cast him out. Exorcising of the devil was the therapy advocated by the priests. The physician of that day wore a long robe or a short fur-edged coat, just as the modern physician wears a white coat. He was usually depicted as holding and gazing at a flask of urine, while the modern physician is portrayed wearing a stethoscope, while a reflecting mirror is strapped to his forehead. The old time doctor believed in astrology and the mystiques attached to amulets, charms, and talismans. He only purged his patients at the most propitious time and performed blood letting at the proper conjunction of the planets. Palmistry was very popular and of course received due consideration.

Paracelsus, of which we will say something very shortly, believed in the "doctrine of signatures". This theory held that a drug bears some supposed resemblance to a particular disease. Therefore a trefoil was good for heart disease, walnut shells for injuries to the head, a thistle for a stitch in the side, turmeric for jaundice, bear's grease for baldness, and, most ridiculous of all, the supposition that ingestion of powdered mummy would prolong life. Very few medical doctors attacked these beliefs. Only a very few surgeons were competent. Charlatanism and quackery were widespread everywhere, and practiced by a motley conglomeration of people such as peddlers, tinkers, horse gelders, leechers, broom men, idiots, bawds, old women, rat-catchers, witches, conjurers, soothsayers, and fortune-tellers.

Another disease which reached epidemic proportions around 1520 was gonorrhea. While this disease was known in antiquity, it had never spread so far and so fast as it did at this period. The reason given was the popularity of the public baths in the cities where both men and women bathed together in one huge vat. Due to the intermingling of the people, sexual excesses resulted, with a breakdown in public morals. As a result, laws were passed segregating the sexes in the baths. Finally, when it became apparent that mass public bathing had something to do with the spread of infection and epidemics, the custom stopped.

Paracelsus (1493-1541) was one of the outstanding physicians of the Renaissance. He was far in advance of his time and rejected Galenisms and the four humors theories. He taught physicians of his day to use chemical therapeutics, instead of alchemy, in prescribing for patients. He castigated witchcraft and the strolling quacks who engaged in surgery as they went from town to town butchering their patients. He attacked and opposed astrology and the stupid urine examinations which were conducted more for their effect on the patients than in actually gathering any useful knowledge. Paracelsus was the first to advocate mineral baths. He made mercury, opium, iron, sulfur, arsenic, copper and potassium sulfate part of the pharmacopeia of his day. He regarded zinc as an elementary substance. In his opinion, living things descended from a primordial mud or ooze. He did not believe in surgery.

Paracelsus wrote some notable treatises. Among these were his works on syphilis, miners' diseases, and mental disorders. The latter two are classics and are considered among the first in their fields. Some historians claim Paracelsus was the father of anaesthesia, for he noted ether had an anesthetic effect on chickens. It is unfortunate such knowledge was not utilized and only came into fruition in the 19th century.

Many authorities have felt that the greatest physician of this age was Vesalius (1514-64). He performed many human dissections and recorded the results in his famous book the *Fabrica*. He completely discredited Galen's animal dissections, when applied to man, and showed that human anatomy has its own succinct features. In the field of physiology, he confirmed a number of Galen's experiments. For example, he showed that artificial respiration would keep an animal alive after the chest had been opened, and that a heart, which had ceased to beat, could be restored to activity by the use of bellows. He also substantiated Galen's findings on the actual functions of muscles and nerves. During Vesalius' lifetime, a physician by the name of Fracastorius developed the theory that micro-organisms caused infections. He did not conceive of them as living bacteria, but as some type of colloids and believed they could reproduce in proper media.

Dissection of human beings had been frowned upon since Roman days. The theologians considered the body holy. After the time of Vesalius, dissections became a bit more popular, were considered as social functions, and required a papal permit. The body or cadaver was duly prepared for dissection by reading the official permit, after which it was stamped with the seal of the university. Then it was taken into the anatomy hall where it was duly decapitated. The head was not utilized because of the popular dislike of opening the brain cavity. After the dissection of the body, there was a celebration with band music or even the presentation of performances at the local theatre. In time, this led to the building of anatomic theatres. It is indeed strange that dissections should be the cause of merrymaking and festive occasions. In 1540, Henry VIII authorized the turning over of four criminal bodies a year for dissection. In 1564, Queen Elizabeth allowed the bodies of two criminals to be utilized each year.

The third great physician of the Renaissance was Ambroise Pare' (1510-90). He was definitely influenced by the work of the great anatomist Vesalius, and made his *Latim Fabrica* popular and understandable to surgeons by writing a summary of it in the common language of the day. Originally a barber, Pare' became an army surgeon, and with his keen observations and discernment he eventually became the greatest surgeon of his time. His famous saying, "I dressed the wound, God healed it," became immortal. Pare's therapy was the complete antithesis of treatment in his day, when wounds, especially after amputations of extremities, were treated with boiling oil and other measures which only encouraged infection and loss of life. Pare' had formerly used boiling oil, and one day after a battle when supplies of oil ran out, he used soothing remedies and noticed that the wounds of these soldiers healed more rapidly and without infection. This incident inspired him to write about his results and to condemn the long accepted and dangerous treatment of wounds.

Pare' invented new surgical instruments and brought back the use of ligatures for tying off blood vessels, a method which had been disregarded since the days of Celsus. He helped to popularize massaging of the body, the use of artificial limbs, and insertion of artificial eyes of silver and gold. He introduced the reimplantation of teeth.

The three great leaders of the Renaissance were Paracelsus, Vesalius, and Pare'. Yet, they were ignored in the universities, and the writings of the ancient physicians were still paramount. With new developments, the 16th century school gradually changed their outlook. The most popular medical schools were Padua; Bologna, and Pisa followed by Paris, Montpelier, and Basel. But now, new universities were being founded at Valencia (1500), Toledo (1518), Jena (1558), Leyden (1577), Edinburgh (1582) and Dublin (1591).

In our modern era, students are demanding a voice in the running of their universities, in the hiring and firing of the faculty, and in passing judgement on the abilities of their teachers. These demands, many feel, represent a new turn in education. Actually, this is not so but is a reversal to medieval times.

Each of the medieval universities were autonomous islands of democracy in the fullest sense. Students elected the rector, professors, and other officers and also determined the courses of study. Elections of the faculty were valid for one year only and then repeated. Naturally, the unpopular teachers were voted out. In those days, there was much camadaderie between professors and students, the faculty wanting to keep on good terms with the students and the students desiring a reciprocal relationship. The two groups often socialized and drank together in the taverns, the students usually paying the bar bill. This was especially true the night before examinations, when the students tried to get the faculty to give them hints on the examination questions.

This system resulted in teachers and students being in a continual flux, moving from one university to another, particularly when the professors were not re-elected or students flunked out. In some cases, the professors moved to other seats of learning to get better jobs and advancement. Students often moved to study under the tutelage of a famous personality.

Many wandering students thus became vagabonds, barely eking out enough for food and lodging, and working at most menial jobs to survive. In many cases they resorted to stealing, thereby bringing down on themselves the anger of the burgomasters, townspeople, and farmers. Fagging and hazing of students was often quite severe. Wild and riotous orgies caused many to drop out and go home as their funds ran out. Yet many applied themselves, even though they were extremely poor, and left the universities to become successful in their chosen careers.

In our present century, we have seen many examples of dancing madness. But for sheer numbers and participation, the Middle Ages far exceeded us with their Dancing Mania. As the Black Death Plague was subsiding, a peculiar epidemic, if we can call it such, broke out in Germany and spread over Europe. It was called St. John's or St. Vitus' dance. Around 1374, large groups of men and women congregated in the streets of Aachen, forming circles, holding hands, and dancing with maniacal frenzy. They danced for hours until exhausted, oblivious of their surroundings, or the jeers and insults of the spectators. Groups of these dancing psychopaths traveled from town to town inducing new recruits to join them. People stopped working everywhere, for the dance was the in-thing. Boys and girls left home, servants left their masters to join in and follow the epidemic beat.

Drugs, Demons, Doctors, and Disease

The disturbed clergy considered this the work of the devil and treated the possessed with exorcism. As in any movement, there are malicious takeovers. Thieves and malcontents joined in with the throngs and soon trouble started. Disorders were put down by the authorities and arrests made. In Strassburg, the authorities divided the revelers into small groups and they were taken to the Chapels of St. Vitus where the priests treated them with religious methods. The widespread epidemic gradually subsided, but occasional outbreaks occurred for several centuries. Paracelsus described them in the 15th century, and, in Italy, cases were noted even in the 16th century, where people believed it was due to tarantula bites.

Another interesting practice in the Middle Ages was the king's touch. Superstition endowed the king with divine healing and great stress was laid upon this miraculous treatment. If he could not deliver, he was considered not legitimate, for God granted to true sovereigns the power to cure everybody. King William of England was the last English king to practice this custom and finally discarded it as a silly superstition.

A most interesting observation of the Middle Ages was the struggle for commercial and sea power. This lasted for over nine centuries, and in the endeavor, power passed from Venice to Lisbon to Amsterdam to London. The struggle was primarily over the huge profits made in the drug traffic. For drugs were the best commercial cargoes to carry. They were light, compact, and the demand was very heavy. More money could be made on these trips than on any others. There was a brisk traffic in drugs like aloes, cloves, benzoin, camphor, cinnamon, cubebs, ginger, musk, mace, nard, nutmeg, opium, pepper, rhubarb, and sandalwood. Ships carried these valuable cargoes from far-away romantic spots such as India, Ceylon, Sumatra, Indo-China, Timor, and China.

Chapter Four

SEVENTEENTH AND EIGHTEENTH CENTURY MEDICINE

THE SEVENTEENTH CENTURY WAS the age of such outstanding men as Shakespeare, Milton, Rembrandt, Cervantes, Spinoza, Galileo, Kepler, Bacon, Descartes, and Locke. It was the time of the Great Armada, the Thirty Years' War, and the advancement of science.

The year beginning the century, 1600, is best remembered for the publication, De Magnete, by William Gilbert, physician to Queen Elizabeth. Overcoming the superstitions about magnetism, Gilbert demonstrated that the earth is a giant magnet and thereby established the true reason for the deflection of the compass needle. His was the prime work for the study of terrestrial magnetism.

The greatest discovery of this century was the disclosure of the circulation of the blood by William Harvey (1578-1657), a graduate of Padua University. The discovery ranks Harvey with Vesalius. This fact was long looking for a discoverer, and many missed it. Galen had considered an ebb and flow theory, and believed that the blood passed from the right side of the heart to the left side of the heart through invisible pores. Vesalius could find no such pores. An Arabian physician, Ibn al Nafis, in the thirteenth century suggested that blood went from the right heart to the lungs to be mixed with air and return to the left heart. The first one to mention this in the West was Servetus, yet this fact remained unnoticed for 144 years until the time of Charles Bernard, an English surgeon. Harvey showed that the heart is a muscular pump which propels the blood in a continuous circle from arteries to veins, back again to the right side of the heart, through the lungs to the left side of the heart, and into the arteries again. What he could not fathom was the connection between the arteries and veins which soon became known through the invention of the microscope.

Harvey's theory of blood circulation was, as usually happens in medicine with any new idea, vigorously opposed. But his experiments convinced his critics gradually that his theory was an absolute fact. However, Harvey's conception of respiration was that of Aristotle, who believed the sole function of breathing was to cool off the blood, an impression that delayed for too long the recognition of the real physiology of breathing.

The development of the microscope actually goes back to antiquity. The Romans were acquainted with lenses for burning, and Seneca stated that letters could be enlarged by being observed through a glass bulb filled with water. An Arabian physicist by the name of Alhazen observed the magnification attained by a lens. Roger Bacon, in the thirteenth century, described a lens to enlarge small objects or reading material. Armati is credited with the invention of eyeglasses in the thirteenth century. The microscope was invented by Johannes Jansen and his son in Holland around 1590. They were spectacle makers and probably found by serendipity that two convex lenses held at the proper distance produced a high magnification. News spread to Italy and the wily Galileo made a microscope in 1624 and then a telescope.

At first, the men of science used the microscope, then later the physicians. Athanasius Kirscher in 1658 reported that "broods of worms" appeared under the microscope in the blood of bubonic plague victims. He was the first to state the cause of infection. Robert Hook (1635-1680), a brilliant physiologist, first described the red cells of the blood. Leeuwenhoek (1637-1723) was the first to note spermatozoa, protozoa, and the capillary connection between arteries and veins, thus completing Harvey's circle of blood movement.

Other discoveries followed. Galileo invented the alcohol thermometer between 1593 and 1597. He considered it a joke and called it in Italian "scherzine," meaning a little joke. Sanctorius (1561-1636) however, realizing its value medically, developed three types of thermometers—a mouth, hand and one into which a patient breathed. He also invented a pulse clock, timing the pulse by a pendulum, and adjusting the length of the cord so that the pendulum swung at the same rate as the pulse beat. The latter was then expressed in terms of the length of the cord. He was also the father of metabolism, weighing himself before and after meals and also his excreta; he realized there was an unaccountable loss which he referred to as insensible perspiration.

Sylvius (1614-72) was the physiological chemist of his time, popularizing Harvey's theories as Pare' had done for Vesalius. He was one of the greatest teachers of his era. He studied acids, salts, and alkalies, being the innovator in explaining the acidosis and alkalosis of disease. He pondered over the function of glands and regarded digestion as being a form of chemical fermentation. His followers, of which there were many, recommended the medical use of large quantities of the newly imported substances, tea and coffee, for treatment of many medical disorders. Willis (1621-75) was one of his famous pupils. He described the diseases of myasthenia gravis, typhoid fever, and puerperal or childbirth fever.

Before Harvey's time, men believed that the purpose of breathing was to cool the fiery heart. Harvey demonstrated that blood changed from venous to arterial after passing through the lungs, but did not know how. Boyle (1627-91) showed that air is necessary for life. Hooke, like Vesalius, kept a dog alive by pumping air with a bellows into its trachea or windpipe, after the lungs were punctured and remained quiescent, proving motion of the lungs was not the essential factor in respiration but rather blood changes.

Richard Lower (1631-91), who was the first to perform blood transfusions between animals, injected dark venous blood into inflated lungs and noted the color became bright, indicating it had absorbed air. Mayow deemed this to be an igneous ingredient of the air. Scientists in the next century found this substance to be oxygen.

During the Renaissance, the physicians usually were interested in several fields besides medicine, notably botany and zoology. In the seventeenth century, the outstanding physicians were often very versatile, being very knowledgeable and teaching several university courses in disciplines other than medicine. Among the physicists-medicos were Descartes, Borelli, Kepler, Hooke, and

Sanctorius. Helmont was the first to use the term "gas." Boyle founded analytic chemistry and discovered Boyle' law which relates to gases and pressure. Redi and Leeuwenhoek were the first food chemists. John Glauber discovered Glauber's salts (sodium sulfate).

Intravenous injections and transfusions of foreign blood began in this century. Christopher Wren, aided by Boyle and Wilkins, injected opium and other drugs into dogs in 1656. Major was the first to inject drugs into humans intravenously. Transfusion of sheep blood into a human was done by Lower between 1665 and 1667.

Sydenham was considered one of the greatest medical men of the seventeenth century. He described scarlet fever, hysteria, and chorea. In his practice, he popularized Peruvian bark (quinine), advised horseback riding for consumptives, cooling liquids for smallpox, iron tonics for anemia, and liquid opiates which were named after him. He also prescribed vegetable materials and avoided the filthy prescriptions of the *London Pharmacopeia* of his time.

A glance at the medications used in the 1618 and 1650 London Pharmacopeias is rather interesting and amusing. Among them were worms, lozenges of dried vipers, oil of bricks, oil of ants, foxes' lungs for asthma, powders made from precious stones, and oil of wolves. Many preparations still had the names of their ancient Greek and Arabic innovator. There were also oddities like moss from the skull of a violently killed person, Gascoyne's powder made of crabs' eyes, black tops of crabs' claws, amber, pearls, bezoar, and Neapolitan (blue) ointment.

A later edition of the *London Pharmacopeia* of 1685 disclosed that the names of the Greek and Arabian formulas were disappearing and more worthy medications were being added such as quinine, jalap (cathartic), alum, digitalis, iron tonics, balsams of tolu, and Irish whiskey. Human urine was highly recommended by Madame de Sevigne at this time.

Among the very unusual remedies in the three editions of the seventeenth century were bones, bile, blood, body organs, claws, hoofs, sex organs, excretions from all types of animals, fur, feathers, human perspiration, spider webs, raw silk, sea shells, snake spins, and wood lice.

The great medical men of these times prescribed some pretty

weird concoctions. Yet we can't be too severe on them, for they were in much the same situation as the ancient Egyptians; they had discovered nothing better. Minderer (discoverer of ammonium acetate) used oil of spiders and earthworms for bubonic plague. For dysentery, Lemery prescribed cat ointment and oil of young puppies boiled together with earthworms. For the same condition, Mattioli preferred oil of scorpions, and Paracelsus prescribed human feces.

The eighteenth century produced the great philosophers Fichte, Kant, Liebnitz, and Hegel. In music, the greats were Bach, Haydn, and Handel. The outstanding writers were Pope, Rousseau, and Voltaire. In the sciences the giants were Cavendish, Laplace, Lagrange, Lavoisier, Priestly, Scheele, Volta, Galvani, Franklin, Fahrenheit, and Watt.

In medicine, according to Fielding, the great medical historian, it was an age of theorists and systematists, a dull period characterized with a scarcity of original thinkers except for men like Hales, Hunter, Morgagni, Jenner, and Wolff. But let us examine this period and draw our own conclusions.

Linnaeus, Swedish Botanist and physician, established the custom of classification in both botany and medicine. He originated the double naming or binominal system in which each natural object received a family or generic name and then a specific or given name. He classified man in the order of Primates and then called him "Homo Sapiens" or wise man.

The outstanding theorist of the eighteenth century was George Ernst Stahl (1660-1734) whose conception of "animism" gained many adherents. According to this theory, the body is a machine directed by the anima or soul. Disease is due to faulty control by the anima. Altered tone and plethora (blood vessel loss of tone) caused pathology (disease). He relieved plethora by frequent and copious bloodletting. He believed that fever was due to overactivity of the anima and should not be reduced as it was beneficial, an opinion still held today by some physicians. He considered opium and quinine harmful. If the anima was not successful in overcoming disease, then he suggested venesection, laxatives, emetics (vomiting agents), and diaphoretic drugs. While Stahl's thinking was retrogressive, he made a valuable contribution in that he emphasized the unity of the living body.

The animism of Stahl became important to the anthropologists and psychiatrists of the nineteenth and early twentieth centuries. In 1871, Taylor employed this theory to explain the psychology of primitive man. As an advocate of psychotherapy, Stahl is a link between present thinking and that of the past. He keenly noted the effects of the mind upon the body and his theory of the distraught psyche as the cause of disease contains beginning elements of the doctrines of Freud. The psychosomatic concepts follow along naturally in these lines, namely the effects of the mind on the body.

The animism of Stahl became merged into the vitalism theory. Johann F. Blumbach (1752-1840), a devoted follower of Stahl, advocated this concept in expressing the idea that an inner impulse or vital principle in living creatures motivates them to reproduction and development. William Cullen (1710-90) theorized that life is a function of nervous energy. The phrase "nerve force" in modern times replaced the old Galenic idea of "animal spirit". In a sense, even today, when a physician says a disorder is nervous, he is probably, unconsciously, referring back to Cullen.

Friedrich Hoffman (1660-1742) believed that an ether-type substance, transmitted through the nervous system, exerted its effect on the muscles, keeping them in a partially constricted state. It also imparted motility to the body humors, thus sustaining life. Acute diseases were due to spasticity or constriction, chronic diseases to atony or relaxation. This idea is similar to the theories of the ancient Methodists, as exemplified by Asclepiades, which stressed strictus and laxus. However, Hoffman also believed that humoral changes and faulty excretion could produce some diseases. These four entities could be remedied by sedatives, tonics, alteratives, and evacuants. According to Allbutt (1900), Hoffman was the first physician to note that pathology is a part of physiology.

John Brown (1735-88) introduced his Brunonian theory. He considered all living tissues as excitable, and life was only existent when external or internal stimuli acted upon them. Diseases were therefore sthenic (strong) or asthenic (weak) depending upon the vital condition or excitement being increased or decreased. Treatment was therefore either stimulation or depression of the disorder. Brown's favorite drugs were wine or opium. His own addiction to these drugs eventually killed him. His ideas were rejected in England and France but accepted in America, Italy and Germany.

Drugs, Demons, Doctors, and Disease

Albert von Haller (1708-77) was one of the ablest physicians of all times. He was a distinguished physiologist and is considered the father of modern physiology. Many of his discoveries were forgotten and later rediscovered. Among them are the myogenic (muscle arising) theory of the origin of the heartbeat and the digestion of fat by the bile.

Among other systematists were Bernardino Ramazzini (1633-1714) who keenly observed different occupational diseases and from these studies came the specialty of occupational diseases. Johann Blumbach (1752-1840) investigated the various human races and his work led to the beginning of modern ethnology. Johann Frank (1745-1821) was the founder of public hygiene and Peter Camper, the founder of anthropolgy and craniology.

Leopold Auenbrugger (1722-1809) made one of the greatest discoveries in chest diagnosis. His father was a tavern keeper, and as a boy he used to tap the wine casks to determine how much wine was still available. He applied this principle to the human chest and as a result the science of percussion or chest tapping was born. So when a doctor taps your chest, to determine evidence of disease, he is using Auenbrugger's method to look for fluid (wet pleurisy), air (pneumothorax from a lung perforation), and thickened tissue (consolidation in pneumonia).

We shall now consider the men of the eighteenth century who were original investigators and contributed to the advancement of medical knowledge. The first of these is Giovanni B. Morgagni (1682-1771) who at the age of 79 published his great life's work in five volumes. He was the first to correlate autopsy findings with clinical findings. He checked the patient's symptoms with the changes seen in the patient's organs after death. Consequently, he laid the solid foundation for modern pathology. He described many new forms of disease. Among these were syphilitic involvement of the brain and heart, acute atrophy of the liver, brain infection following ear infection. He also noted that, in strokes, the brain blood vessel affected was always on the opposite side to the paralyzed side. If the left side of the body was paralyzed the blood vessel responsible was on the right side of the brain.

Stephen Hales (1677-1761), an English clergyman, was an inventive genius. He originated artificial respiration in 1743. He investigated the movement of sap in plants. He was the first man to devise a method of taking blood pressure. He inserted a glass tube inside a horse's artery and registered the blood pressure by the height to which it rose, estimated the capacity of the heart's output, and calculated the velocity of the circulation. His researches were far in advance of his time.

John Hunter (1728-93) was the founder of modern surgery. Until his time, the French were the leading surgeons; however, they knew nothing about pathology. It was said by his contemporaries that he found surgery a mechanical art and left it an experimental science. Surgeons after his time were no longer ignorant barbers practicing surgery. His dissections were most extensive in both man and animals. His writings were most prodigious and based upon his own personal research. He left over 13,000 specimens in his great museum. He introduced artificial feeding through a flexible tube inserted into the stomach. He invented an apparatus for forced artificial respiration among his many innovations.

Edward Jenner (1794-1823) was a pupil of John Hunter and helped him in many of his experiments. As a result, he became a shrewd observer. He noted that milkmaids who had contracted cowpox never developed smallpox. He then used cowpox pus to prevent smallpox and published a paper on his results in 1798, and was both attacked and praised. News of the success of this treatment rapidly spread all over Europe and America, and Jenner carved an immortal niche for himself in the annals of medicine. His discovery wiped out forever the scarred faces of men and women who survived a natural attack of smallpox. While he was not the first to try inoculation (others used dried smallpox pus), he was the first to put it on a scientific basis. Jenner was well ahead of his time and the first to demonstrate prophylactic or preventive immunization against a disease. No further virus vaccine was available until the twentieth century when, in World War II, flu virus vaccine was introduced. Jenner's discovery was one of the greatest in the history of medicine, saving millions of lives every year.

While it is not generally realized, Jenner was aware of angina pectoris (suffocating chest pain) previously described by Heberden, and recognized its gravity in their mutual friend, John Hunter. Jenner's dissection experience in autopsies on angina patients made him aware of the thickening of the coronary arteries of the heart and the plaque formation in these vessels. He wrote a paper on the subject.

Drugs, Demons, Doctors, and Disease

The treatment of scurvy in the eighteenth century was unsatisfactory. John Pringle thought it was due to putrid causes in marshy country. However, sailors on long cruises developed the disease. Jacques Cartier, while in Canada in 1556, was in danger of losing his entire crew from scurvy. He heard about an Indian remedy for scurvy consisting of an extract made from either sassafras or spruce tree. He gave this preparation to his crew and they were cured in six days. This scourge decimated armies and navies. James Lind (1716-94), a navy surgeon, discovered that lemon juice would cure and prevent the condition. He recorded his observations and noted, in his paper on the Treatment of Scurvy, that others in the 16th and 17th centuries had used citrous products for scurvy. Lind later recommended oranges and limes. Several of his friends in the navy adopted his treatment with success. But it was 41 years after he had published his paper that the British Admiralty finally ordered lemon juice to be given to the crews on all warships. Lind also wrote a paper on "Jail Fever." He was aware of the fact that this (typhus) fever was transmitted by clothing and suggested that the clothing of such patients and their bedding be destroyed. He cited case studies to prove his point.

One interesting practitioner of this century was George Baker (1722-1809) of London. He investigated a colicky condition that was common in Devon but rare in Hereford. He found that Devon farmers used lead-lined cider presses, while the farmers of Hereford did not. In the cider from Devon, he could demonstrate lead, but not in Hereford cider. When he publicized this fact, he was fiercely attacked by the Devon populace, and branded a traitor to his native soil. However, when the Devon farmers got rid of their lead liners, the Devon cider provoked no more colic. Baker was, therefore, and not an early detector of lead poisoning.

William Withering (1741-1799), a native of Shropshire, was a very busy practitioner and an avid student of botany. He bought a secret remedy from an old woman in Shropshire which cured dropsy. The formula was made up of 20 or more herbs. Withering finally decided that the purple foxglove was the active ingredient. From its leaves comes digitalis, one of the great drugs for treating heart failure or cardiac dropsy. Withering' disclosure of digitalis' value in medicine rates with the great discoveries.

Caleb Parry (1755-1822) published one of the earliest accounts on angina pectoris which he shrewdly attributed to coronary artery disease. His posthumously published papers contained the first lucid account of exophthalmic (eye protrusion) goitre.

Let us now examine the pharmacopeia of the eighteenth century and see if there had been any progress made since the seventeenth century. The fourth pharmacopeia of 1721 omitted many of the old syrups and waters, but retained excreta and other products of animals. Newly introduced was stramonium (relaxant) gamboge (cathartic), ipecac (emetic), lime water, secale cornutum (ergot), liver, inorganic chemicals, tartar emetic. The fifth London pharmacopeia of 1746 was revised by several outstanding medical authorities who condemned the old folk and astrologic medications. While it dropped some ridiculous preparations such as spider webs, moss from human skulls, human fat, and virgin's milk, it still contained such items as vipers, wood lice, crab eyes, and pearls. New tinctures were added such as cardamon (flatulence reliever or carminative) and valerian (tonic), also incorporated were sweet spirits of nitre (diaphoretic, antispasmodic), potassium acetate, and syrup of squills (expectorant).

Due to the persistent attacks of Heberden on the ludicrous preparations in the pharmacopeia, the sixth London edition of 1788 dropped out all animal medications. New drugs added were castor oil, arnica (skin irritant), aconite (cold aborter), cascarilla (tonic), quassia (fever reducer), kino (astringent), magnesia, ether, zinc oxide, tincture of opium, tincture of opium and camphor (paregoric), sarsaparilla. Among some of the interesting preparations were Dover's powders (opium and ipecac), even used in this century. They were a diaphoretic mixture, compounded by Thomas Dover a pirate physician who incidentally rescued Alexander Selkirk (Robinson Crusoe) from the island of Juan Fernandes. Digitalis did not appear until the publication of the pharmacopeia of 1809, although Withering announced it in 1785. Thomas Fowler introduced his arsenic solution in 1786, which was named after him as Fowler's solution, and this preparation is used also in the twentieth century for asthma. Hoffman, whom we have mentioned earlier, discovered a mineral spring in Seidlitz, in Czechoslovakia, from which came the name Seidlitz powders, formerly a popular American headache remedy.

The diseases of an epidemic nature were more scattered than in former years, in the eighteenth century. Among these were scarlet fever, influenza, diphtheria, whooping cough, malaria, and typhus fever. Plague, syphilis, and ergotism were less severe. Infant mortality was very high. Babies, which were not nursed, died at the rate of three to one compared to nursed babies. The earliest substitutes for mother's milk were boiled bread or baked flour mixed with water to make a pap. Sometimes sugar was added. Frequently, this regimen was followed by regular bread, turtle doves, and beer. Artificial feeding began in this century. Michael Underwood in 1784 came out with his formula consisting of boiled cow's milk, diluted with barley water. Soft foods added were tapioca, rice, or semolina. The original nursing bottle was a cow's horn. Then came the glass bottle, the pap boat, and the pap spoon. The nipple was originally parchment, then leather, sponge, a young cow's teats, or it was fashioned from wood or india rubber.

Stephen Hales, the scientific genius and clergyman, conducted experiments in fermentation and distillation. His main interest was in the gaseous property of solids, rather than in the nature and properties of the gases themselves. His work came to the attention of other investigators who were interested in the properties and nature of the gases primarily.

Black discovered carbon dioxide in 1757, Cavendish isolated hydrogen in 1766. Rutherford discovered nitrogen in 1772. Priestley and Scheele discovered oxygen in 1771 and Lavoisier confirmed it in 1775.

Lavoisier was the first to understand that respiration was oxidation and that expired air contained carbon dioxide. He believed that body respiration took place in the lungs, but this erroneous impression was corrected by Spallanzani and others who showed that all tissues respire, taking up oxygen and giving off carbon dioxide. As a result of the discovery of oxygen, some physicians undertook to treat all diseases with this gas, believing that diseases are either due to a lack of or an excess of oxygen. In 1798, Beddoes opened a Pneumatic Institute for treating diseases by inhalations of this gas. James Watt, the inventor of the steam engine and radiator, constructed the apparatus for Beddoes and also invented the gasometer. Beddoes' assistant in this treatment was Humphrey Davey, who discovered the anaesthetic properties of nitrous oxide. Beddoes and Watt developed the idea of treating respiratory diseases with inhalations of various gases. The modern use of oxygen therapy was initiated by these men.

During the eighteenth century, interesting developments occurred in the field of electricity. In antiquity, certain electrical phenomena had been discovered by the ancient Greeks. They knew that when amber was stroked or rubbed it had certain attracting powers; it became electrified. In fact, our word for electricity comes from the Greek word for amber. In the sixteenth century, Queen Elizabeth's physician, William Gilbert, who wrote a monumental work on magnetism, explained the power of attraction as an electrical force. In the seventeenth century Boyle, Newton, and Guericke, inventor of the air pump, conducted many electrical experiments. In the eighteenth century, Hauksbee used electricity to produce light. Gray demonstrated that electrical attraction was transferable from one body to another. The Leyden jar was discovered. Benjamin Franklin showed that electricity and lightening were the same, using his famous kite experiment. Galvani, employing electrical currents, noted that they caused muscular contractions in animals. Caldani used electrical stimulation upon the cortex of the brain.

Galvani (1737-98), went further in his experimentation and showed that excised frog muscles in contact with two dissimilar metals would go into spasms. Alessandro Volta (1745-1827) followed up these experiments and developed the Voltaic pile, known as the electric battery.

As with oxygen, physicians and non-professionals immediately began to employ this new modality for all kinds of medical purposes. Benjamin Franklin used electricity to treat diseases, especially paralysis. John Wesley, the Methodist evangelist, used it to treat his parishioners' ailments. DeHaen of Vienna believed that he cured St. Vitus dance with electricity. The fanatical electric adherents utilized this method for treatment and alleged cure of almost anything. London hospitals installed static machines to treat disease. They became very popular and were widely used in Europe and America, and this form of treatment survived until the early years of the twentieth century.

One of the most interesting characters of this age was Franz Anton Mesmer, (1734-1815) whose name is synonymous with mesmerism. He first studied theology and philosophy, later going to Vienna to become a physician. He believed that the planets influence the tissues of the human body, through a mysterious fluid which he called animal magnetism. He backed up this theory by quoting physicians in the past who believed in the influence of the heavenly bodies on human behavior and disease. In 1777, while in Vienna, he claimed to have cured a patient, blind since the age of three. He was so violently attacked by the local physicians that he fled to Paris.

When in Paris, Mesmer built up a huge following of neurotic, wealthy patients, while earning the enmity of the medical profession. He built a magnetic chamber, in which the patients sat around a large tub from which protruded iron bars. The patients joined hands together, thus completing a circle around the tub. Mesmer then appeared, dressed in a purple robe and carrying a magic wand. Moving about slowly he would touch one of the group with his wand. The person began to twitch, gyrate, and turn and then the whole group began to react similarly. These crises, as Mesmer called them, had to occur before the animal magnetism could cure. King Louis XVI appointed a committee of the Academy of Sciences, which included Benjamin Franklin and Lavoisier, to investigate this treatment. They concluded, after using an electrometer and a compass, that there was no magnetism involved, and that the patients' reactions were wholly due to their "vivid imaginations." Mesmer continued to prosper despite this adverse report. The French revolution finally drove him from Paris and he fled to Switzerland where he eventually died. Mesmer was not an actual swindler but sincerely believed in his theory of animal magnetism. Tischner considered Mesmer a second rate intellectual who misunderstood what he had discovered, namely mesmerism.

Puysegur, a disciple of Mesmer, while working with mesmerism rediscovered hypnotism. Mesmerism soon became synonymous with hypnotism. This new treatment quickly spread all over Europe and even to America. In America, Phineas Quimby, who founded the cult of New Thought and used mesmerism or hypnosis, concluded that the healing power was actually the faith of the patient. Among his patients was Mary Baker Eddy who later founded her own cult known as Christian Science. Mesmerism also gave rise to Unity, Cueism, and other groups. Hypnotism is employed extensively today in diagnostic and therapeutic approaches to the functional neuroses. Psychoanalysis is closely related to hypnosis, or what was formerly known as artificial somnabulism or mesmerism.

Quackery naturally flourished in this age when the most that

Drugs, Demons, Doctors, and Disease

could be given patients were pukes (emetics), purges, and bloodletting. No doubt these heroic measures made the patients feel worse than their diseases. Many were probably killed by these procedures. As physicians had no cures for the common maladies, people looked for help elsewhere. With the exception of digitalis and quinine, there were no specific remedies for disease. Enemas, called clysters, were a very highly regarded form of treatment. Louis XIV of France had two thousand enemas during his lifetime. Fashionable ladies even took enemas while attending the theatre. Bleeding was so popular that, in one year, thirty three million leeches were imported into France. Between bloodletting and leeching, more blood was shed in European countries by these methods than all their wars.

Among the most famous quacks of this period was Joshua Ward. He was originally a salt dryer. But he became famous for his antimony pills, a liquid sweat, a powder for purging dropsy, a headache essence, and his very famous paste for piles. Ward made a fortune selling these products. His fame reached the king and he was invited to court, where he soon mixed in the highest aristocratic circles.

Favorite medical fads of these times were quassia cups, saffron drops, cathartic sugar plums, special anodyne necklaces made to be worn by pregnant mothers and teething children, Perkins' magnetic tractors for drawing disease out of the body.

James Graham, a Scotsman, opened a "Temple of Health" in London in 1780. This was a luxuriously appointed affair. Here he undertook to cure sterility and impotency on his famous "Celestial Beds." These beds were highly perfumed and musical, and while the occupants were engaged in love making, animal magnetism and electrical currents were supposedly applied to increase the vigor of the love makers. Emma Lyon, the future Lady Hamilton, was the high priestess of this cult. Again, treatment was mesmerism or self-hypnosis. The business finally failed, and Graham turned next to mud-bath quackery which proved to be financially also a debacle.

Hygienic conditions were as bad in this century as in the previous one. This, of course, helped to spread disease. Amusingly, as a sidelight, women's wigs were provided with inserts of honey and vinegar to attract the lice. People stank and perfumes were used to mask the odors. Madame Pompadour boldly made the statement that even the kings stank.

Hospitals of the eighteenth century were horrible, filthy, and a detriment to life. Contagious patients were kept next to non-contagious ones, thus promoting the spread of infection.

The care of the insane was even worse. They were treated like animals, being chained and caged. Harmless ones were allowed to run loose. The noisy atmosphere of the Bedlam Insane Asylum in London gave rise to the word "bedlam" in our language. Curiosity seekers frequented the asylums and were allowed to view the inmates for kicks, paying a small fee for the privilege. Perhaps they were the same people who frequented public hangings for sadistic thrills.

Insanity was considered to be an incurable disorder well into the nineteenth century. Even worse, it was regarded as a disgrace to both the individual and his family. Many believed it to be divine punishment for personal guilt or sin. Insanity, now known by the euphemism of mental illness, was considered by some physicians to be due to disturbances in the yellow or black bile; others felt it was caused by excessive summer heat, vanity, jealousy, envy, or masturbation.

If the afflicted person did not respond to drugs, the physician considered his case hopeless. Melancholy patients were treated with opium, while manic patients received camphor. Belladonna was the last hope and final drug used and if this failed. no further medications were utilized. Among bizarre treatments used were the giving of mixtures of honey and vinegar or large quantities of tepid water, the application to the forehead of plasters made of either Spanish Fly or mustard, the administration of enemas and finally bloodletting from the forehead and thumbs. A woman suffering from depression might be subjected to curses and cold water douches. Manic patients often were given emetics and purgatives to wear them out. If this failed, they were savagely beaten and bound in chains.

A few efforts were made to treat these unfortunate people humanely. They were occasionally put to work in the fields, given animals to care for, or sent to mineral baths. In 1794, the Quaker, William Tuke, set up the first institute at York, England, to provide kind and considerate measures for treating insane patients. Phillippe Pinel of France, in 1798, received permission from the National

Drugs, Demons, Doctors, and Disease

Assembly to free 49 patients from their chains at the insane asylum at Bicetre so that he might try humane therapy instead of drugging and bleeding these unfortunate individuals.

Chapter Five

THE NINETEENTH CENTURY

With the exception of our own century, the nineteenth century was the most remarkable in history both in science and medicine. The exciting advances of our time were built upon the strong foundations laid in the last century. Historically, it was an age of political growth, turmoil, and some measure of stability. It was a time of changing economic patterns, social upheavals, the industrial revolution, and the formative years for socialism and communism.

Politically, in Europe, it was the age of Napoleon, Bismarck, and Queen Victoria. In the Orient, Japan was emerging as a world power. In the United States, there was rapid growth and expansion along with a series of wars with Britain, Mexico, Spain, and between the states.

Great advances were made in the sciences, utilizing the knowledge acquired during the seventeenth and eighteenth centuries.. By the end of the eighteenth century, steam had been harnessed to produce a workable steam engine. In 1804, a steam locomotive was devised and in 1825 George Stephenson built a commercially successful vehicle. In 1807, Robert Fulton sailed the first successful steamboat. Humphrey invented the carbon arc lamp in 1809. In 1822, Michael Faraday constructed an electric motor and, in 1831, produced the electric dynamo. The year 1837 saw Samuel Morse's telegraph. Mayer and Joule proposed the principle of the conservation of energy in 1842 and this knowledge was applied to chemistry and physics by Helmholtz in 1847.

Among important inventions of the century, were the ice machine of Jacob Perkins in 1834, the bicycle of Kirkpatrick MacMillan in 1840, the open hearth furnace of the Siemens brothers for making steel in 1851, the passenger elevator of Elisha Otis in 1857, the typewriter of Sholes, Glidden, and Soule in 1867, the vacuum cleaner of Ives McGaffery in 1869, the telephone of Alexander Bell and the four-cycle engine of Nikolaus Otto in 1876, the electric lamp of Thomas Edison and the cash register of James Ritty in 1879, the electric street car of Werner Siemens in 1881, the electric fan of Henry Seeley and the electric iron of Schuyler Wheeler in 1882, the automobile of Karl Benz and the dictaphone of Charles Tainer in 1885, the motion picture projector of Thomas Edison in 1891, the diesel engine of Rudolph Diesel in 1892, the electric locomotive in 1895, the radio telegraph of Guglielmo Marconi in 1896 (based upon the discovery of radio waves by Heinrich Hertz in 1887) and the electric stove of William Hadaway in the same year.

Other interesting advances were made in this century. Bunsen and Kirschhoff discovered spectral analysis in 1859. Faraday in 1821 and Maxwell in 1864 developed the theories of electricity and electromagnetics from which came electric lighting, the telephone, telegraph, radio, and eventually television. Because of his pioneering work between 1872 and 1878, Josiah Gibbs of Yale University, one of America's most brilliant scientists and relatively unknown today, is responsible for the development of thermodynamics.

Photography dated from the discovery in 1727 by Johann Schultz who noted that silver nitrate darkens in sunlight. Then came Nichephore Niepce in 1811, who made the world's first photograph on a pewter plate, a rather fuzzy picture. The first successful photos were achieved by Louis Daguerre in 1839, utilizing sensitive copper plates treated with mercury vapor. Around 1840, Fox Talbot invented chloride paper film from which copies could be made of the same photo, unlike the daguerreotypes. Scott Archer obsoleted these processes with his wet emulsion plates in 1851. In 1871, Richard Maddox improved upon this method with his dry, more sensitive plates. In 1889, Henry Reichenbach, working for George Eastman of the Kodak Company, invented the roll film. The elements of color photography began in the nineteenth century with the work of James Maxwell and a nephew of Niepce.

Drugs, Demons, Doctors, and Disease

Physicians, who were scientists also, made notable contributions. Thomas Young in 1801 described astigmatism of the eye, in 1802 formulated the wave theory of light, and in 1805 announced the capillary theory of surface tension. John Dalton in 1803 proclaimed the atomic theory. Between 1797 and 1801 William Wolloston studied the chemistry of kidney stones, theorized about stereochemistry, and invented the camera lucida. Helmholtz, in 1850, invented the ophthalmoscope for looking into the interior of the living eye and he also formulated theories on optics and vision.

Most discoveries in the medical field came in the second half of the century. Up to 1850 and well beyond, the French were paramount in the medical profession, then German medicine began its ascendancy. The British and American contributions came in descriptive analyses of disease and the discovery of anesthesia in 1847.

The early part of the century was the era of Napoleon. His invasion into Russia was accompanied by typhus and typhoid epidemics which struck his army when he entered Poland. Failure to control these diseases, according to Kerckhoffs, a Dutch army surgeon in Napoleon's army, cost him the Russian campaign. Upon the retreat of the Grand Army from Russia, typhus and typhoid diseases were disseminated by the troops throughout central Europe. Previous conquests of the French army also spread various epidemics about Europe.

Napoleon's greatest army surgeon was Dominique Larrey, who lived from 1766 to 1842. He was the first one to describe trench foot and also recognize the contagious nature of an Egyptian eye disorder known as the Egyptian ophthalmia. Larry used a flexible catheter to feed soldiers who received neck wounds and were unable to swallow food. He also originated the so-called "flying ambulances" which picked up wounded soldiers as soon as a battle began, instead of waiting for it to end, thereby saving many lives.

Rene Laennec (1781-1826) invented the stethoscope in 1816. He watched two children playing with a wooden stick and taking turns listening to their end while the other child tapped at the opposite end. He tried this himself and noted that sound traveled through the wood. He tried the same experiment with a rolled up piece of paper and then repeated it using a hollowed out cylinder of wood. This became the first stethoscope. Placed against the chest it transmitted sounds from the heart and lungs. Thus began the science of auscultation or listening and Laennec wrote the first book on this new development. As the sounds from the chest had never been heard in this fashion before, a new nomenclature was devised by Laennec to describe what he heard. Auscultation was very quickly adopted by physicians, unlike percussion, which was unused by the medical profession for 47 years after Auenbrugger's announcement.

Laennec utilized, in addition to auscultation, the standard methods of physical examination such as inspection, palpation (use of hands in diagnosis), and percussion. In his two books, the first published in 1819 and the second in 1826, Laennec described the physical and autopsy findings in pneumonia, lung cysts, emphysema (destruction of lung tissue), lung embolic phenomena (clot break-offs in blood vessels which travel to the lungs), tuberculosis, pleurisy, and edema of the lungs (waterlogging due to lung circulatory failure caused by a failing heart), and gangrene. In addition to lung diseases, Laennec wrote about heart disorders and described heart murmurs heard through his stethoscope. He also described a cirrhosis of the liver, which was named after him, and is known as Laennec's cirrhosis (a shrinkage and scarring of the liver).

Pierre Bretonneau (1771-1864) described and gave diptheria its present name. In addition, he differentiated between typhoid and tuberculous ulcers of the intestines.

Jean Bouillard (1796-1881) on the basis of clinical and autopsy findings stated that the center for speech is located in the anterior or frontal portion of the brain, confirming the claim of Franz Gall. He gave the name "endocardium" to the lining of the heart and introduced this term, and also "endocarditis," into medicine. The latter term refers to an inflammation of the heart lining. Bouillard saw that, in this condition, there was an exudate on the heart valves which later caused valvular scarring, contracture, and back-leakage of blood with each heart beat. He noted, too, the relationship between endocarditis and rheumatism, which we now call rheumatic fever. He described various abnormal rhythms of the heart. Bouillard was considered an early cardiologist and a prime investigator in his chosen field. Pierre Louis (1781-1872) wrote the most complete and exhaustive work on tuberculosis. His work on typhoid fever in 1829 gave this disease its present name.

Jean Cruveilhier (1791-1874) published a colored atlas of pathology in which, for the first time, there were descriptions and illustrations of disseminated or multiple sclerosis, progressive muscular atrophy, and stomach or gastric ulcer (still called, by the

Drugs, Demons, Doctors, and Disease

French, Cruveilhier's disease). The illustrations and artistry of this great work have never been equaled.

Modern dermatology (study of skin diseases) dates from the work of Robert Wilan (1757-1812) and his pupil Thomas Bateman (1778-1821). Wilan tried to clarify the nature of eczema and lupus (tuberculosis) disease of the skin. He classified skin diseases according to their appearances such as papules (pimples), squamous (scaling), vesicles (blisters), macules (flat appearances), pustular (pus containing elevations) and others. His book on skin diseases described and pictured common skin disorders such as prurigo (an itching skin condition), pityriasis (a scaling skin disease), and ichthyosis (rought scaly skin condition, also known as fish skin disease because of its resemblance to fish scales). He clearly defined impetigo (a pustular skin condition), tinea versicolor (a fungus disease of varying color), sycosis (disease of the hair follicles, especially of the beard), and psoriasis (many believe this was the leprosy described in the Bible afflicting Gehazi and Naaman), which is a silvery scaling condition of the skin. Wilan also described contact dermatitis (inflamed skin) due to external sources of irritation. Bateman published Wilan's unfinished work in an atlas of 72 colored plates in 1817. Bateman was the first physician to describe lichen urticatus (hive-like pimples), molluscum contagiosum (firm elevations of a contagious nature, viral in origin) and ecthyma (an infectious condition of the legs and arms).

Jean-Louis Alibert (1768-1837) was the founder of the French dermatological school. He introduced the term "syphilides" (any eruption due to syphilis), "dermatoses" (skin diseases), and other terms. This phase of descriptions was later followed by von Hebra and other dermatologists who undertook microscopic studies of skin disorders.

Medical experimentation and investigation began early in the century with the work of Francois Magendie (1783-1855). He was an experimental physiologist and studied the mechanics of vomiting and swallowing, the workings of the gastrointestinal (stomach and intestine) tract, the functioning of the cerebellum of the brain, blood circulation and heart beat. His experiments convinced him that indiscriminate bleeding of the patients was foolish and in fact hazardous. In pharmacology, he investigated the drugs morphine, iodine, bromine, emetine, brucine, and veratrine. In 1839, he showed that a rabbit which tolerated one injection of egg white (albumin) frequently died after a second injection. This was the first observation on the phenomenon of anaphylaxis (allergy). One of his early publications in 1822 showed proof that the anterior nerves (which come off the front of the spinal column) are motor nerves while the posterior nerves (that come off the back of the spinal column) carry sensation. The priority of this discovery was disputed by the anatomist Charles Bell (1774-1842) who deducted the same facts from his anatomical investigations. Bell also described Bell's Palsy, a common paralysis of one side of the face due to involvement of the facial nerve.

At about this time, there appeared in Ireland a small group of physicians who left their mark on medical history and were known as the Irish School. Abraham Colles (1773-1843) of Dublin wrote an important paper in 1814 on the fracture of the radius bone of the wrist, and this fracture has been known ever since as Colles' fracture. He also wrote a paper on his observations of the treatment of syphilis with mercury. John Cheyne (1777-1836) of Dublin described hydrocephalus ("water on the brain") in 1808 and Cheyne-Stokes respiration in 1818. This type of breathing is seen especially in coma, and is characterized by rhythmic increasing and then decreasing depth of breathing followed by short periods of no breathing. Then the cycle repeats itself.

William Stokes (1804-1878) of Dublin wrote the first English book on the use of the stethoscope in 1825, an excellent book on diseases of the chest in 1847, and a book on diseases of the heart and aorta in 1854. In the latter, he mentions Cheyne-Stokes respiration, attacks of recurring fast heart beat known as paroxymal tachycardia, and Stokes-Adams disease. The latter condition was first described by Adam in 1827 and is characterized by sudden attacks of unconsciousness or convulsions due to a very slow heart rate caused by heart block due to coronary artery disease.

Dominic Corrigan's (1802-1880) name is associated with "Corrigan's pulse," which he described in 1832 in cases of aortic valvular disease of the heart. This is a jerky pulse with full expansion followed by a sudden collapse. William Wallace (1791-1837) introduced the use of potassium iodide in syphilis. Francis Rynd (1801-1861) introduced his method of giving hypodermic injections to relieve pain by a gravity mechanism.

Robert Graves (1797-1853) of Dublin was very much interested in fevers and opposed the restriction of food which was then the accepted treatment. He, on the contrary, fed fevers. Graves' disease, exophthalmic goitre (overactive thyroid gland with protrusion of the eyeballs), is named after him, although it was mentioned previously by Caleb Parry.

Next we come to the great physicians of Guy's Hospital in London. Richard Bright (1789-1858) was the most famous British physician of his time. He was immortalized for his work on the kidneys, and Bright's disease is named after him. In this condition the blood protein, albumin, leaks through the kidneys into the urine, there is edema or swelling of the tissues, and eventual scarring of the kidneys. Bright also noted that enlargement of the heart and uremia could accompany the kidney condition. Thomas Addison's (1793-1860) name was given to the disease he described, namely, melasma suprarenals, now known as Addison's disease. In this condition, the skin is bronze and there is dysfunction of the suprarenal or adrenal glands. Also named after him is Addison's anemia or pernicious anemia. Addison also noted and described xanthoma diabeticorum (fatty patches found on the skin in some cases of diabetes). Thomas Hodgkin (1798-1866) observed and reported acute appendicitis in 1839. He is, however, famous for his description of Hodgkin's disease, a type of cancer involving the lymph nodes, the spleen, and other lymphatic tissue in the body.

James Parkinson (1755-1824) is best remembered today for his classic description of Parkinson's disease in 1817, a disorder also known as the shaking palsy. Besides practicing medicine, he was interested in fossils and was considered an able geologist and paleontologist.

Samuel Hahnemann (1755-1843) of Germany, introduced the concept of homeopathy. He believed disease could be destroyed by a drug that produces the same disease symptoms, his motto being that "likes cure likes." While his theory enjoyed some popularity for a time, it was eventually discarded. However, Hahnemann's attacks on the employment of strong emetics and cathartics, bleedings, cuppings, and blisterings met with some success. His own medicines, given in very dilute doses, probably did no harm, in contrast to the strong medications used by his contemporaries and antagonists.

An early contributor to hay fever knowledge was John Bostock who described this disorder in 1819. John Elliotson (1791-1868) in 1831 believed that pollen was the cause of hay fever.

Jan Purkinje was the first to use a microtome, an instrument for cutting small slices of tissues. In doing so, he discovered the sweat glands of the skin, and the Purkinje cells of the cerebellum. He observed the identity of animal and plant cells as well as the value of finger prints, long before Francis Galton. He studied carefully the physiology of vision and described the visual images produced in humans by overdoses of digitalis and belladonna. He investigated drugs like opium, camphor, belladonna and turpentine. He also introduced the word "protoplasm" for the living substance of cells.

The first American physician in colonial New England was Samuel Fuller, who served the colony from the landing of the Pilgrims in 1620 until his death in 1633 from smallpox. For a century thereafter, no prominent physician was noted in Massachusetts. According to the historian Viets, medicine was practiced during this period by three classes of people—1) the governors, 2) ordained ministers, and 3) minor physicians, preachers and schoolmasters. Occasionally, British physicians emigrated to the colonies. But, as a rule, young men apprenticed themselves to practicing doctors and eventually opened up their own practices. None attended medical school.

The first American medical school was founded in Philadelphia in 1765 by the University of Pennsylvania at the urging of Dr. John Morgan (1735-1789), who trained both here and abroad. He was appointed the director and so became the first professor of medicine in America. During the revolution, he was also appointed the first surgeon general of the American army. His antagonist and colleague was the obstetrician and anatomist William Shippen, Jr. (1736-1808). Of all the Revolutionary War period physicians, Benjamin Rush (1746-1813) was the most famous. He studied under Morgan and Shippen and then went abroad. He became a follower of Cullen, then of Brown. Consequently, he believed that all diseases were due to debility, which caused excessive irritability. Fever was, therefore, due to blood vessel irritability and so he treated it with a low food intake, purging, and bleeding.

During the yellow fever epidemics in Philadelphia between 1793-1797, Rush treated patients with this regimen, claiming a high cure rate, while his opponents insisted his results were very poor. Rush wrote a number of books and articles. In these, he described vividly the yellow fever epidemics in Philadelphia, the relationship between tooth abscesses and arthritis, the spread of smallpox

Drugs, Demons, Doctors, and Disease

and venereal disease to the Indians by Europeans. Rush was the first American physician to describe cholera, dengue, dropsy, tuberculosis and epidemics of scarlet fever and influenza. He wrote the first American textbook on psychiatry and this remained the only book on the subject in America for about seventy years. In this book, Rush advocated humane treatment for the insane and suggested moderate exercise, diets, and baths for these patients.

The second American medical college was organized in 1768 in New York City. This later became known as Columbia Medical School. Harvard Medical School was the third medical college and was established in 1783. One of its first professors, and a distinguished physician, was Dr. Benjamin Waterhouse. He introduced smallpox vaccination into America in 1800 when he fearlessly inoculated his own son. He then vaccinated other people and, after seeing the excellent results from this therapy, he published the first American medical paper on the subject. Waterhouse was violently attacked by the medical profession for engaging in this daring work and, as a result of this castigation, he lost most of his practice, had to resign his teaching post at Harvard, and suffered severe financial loss and humility.

Ephraim McDowell (1771-1830) performed the first operation in the United States in 1809 to remove an ovarian tumor which, incidentally, weighed out at 22 pounds. The surgery was done on the doctor's kitchen table, took 28 minutes, and no anesthesia was given. The woman survived, and lived for another 33 years, reaching the age of 78. The operation was known as an ovariotomy and Rush, because of this spectacular feat, was called the father of ovariotomy.

William Beaumont (1785-1853), an ex-army surgeon, became one of America's most famous physiologists. In 1822, he treated a Canadian fur trapper, Alexis St. Martin, who had received a gunshot wound in the stomach. When the wound healed, a gaping opening was left in the stomach and so Beaumont could observe digestion in the human stomach, a phenomenon never before witnessed by man. Beaumont took advantage of this unique opportunity to study digestion. He noted what happened to different types of foods placed in the stomach and also what transpired in vials of food into which he placed the gastric juice. He soon became convinced that the old theories on digestion were wrong and that digestion was not due to fermentation or maceration but rather

Drugs, Demons, Doctors, and Disease

to some substance in the gastric juice which dissolved the foods. With the help of a chemist, it was shown that hydrochloric acid was the acid of the stomach; the other substance was shown to be an enzyme, called pepsin, by Theodore Schwann in 1835. Beaumont stated in his published work in 1833 that gastric juice secretions and gastric movements were halted when his patient became angry, thus demonstrating the effects of emotions on the stomach.

McDowells' and Beaumont's accomplishments surprised European doctors, for they considered Americans to be wild frontiersmen and primitive people. Another surprise was soon forthcoming from America.

The next great American contribution to medicine was the introduction of anesthesia for surgical operations. The idea of "putting a patient to sleep," so that he would not feel any pain, was not new. Dioscorides, the great Greek physician of the first century, recommended drinking wine of madragora before surgery. The ancient Hindus used hemp, the Chinese employed hashish, the South American Indians took cocaine or datura (stramonium). The Hindus were also supposed to have had some form of inhalation anesthetic, but we do not know what it was. The Arabians used the soporific or sleep producing sponge which was also recommended by Magister Salernus at the Salerno medical school in the twelfth century. The ancients originated the soporific sponge. This was a sponge impregnated with opium, hyoscyamus, hemlock, and mandragora and allowed to dry. When used, it was dipped in water and then placed over the nose for the patient to breath deeply until he fell asleep. After surgery, a vinegar-soaked sponge placed over the nose would awaken the patient.

Surgeons from the Renaissance period up to 1846 performed operations without any anesthesia. Velpeau, the great French surgeon, said in 1839 that to escape pain in surgery was a chimera not to be expected. Humphrey Davy breathed nitrous oxide in 1798 and noticed its pain relieving effects and suggested its use in surgery. Henry Hickman noted the analgesic or pain relieving effects of breathing carbon dioxide in 1824, but was unable to get surgeons to try this gas.

Ether was synthesized in 1540 by Valerius Cordus. In the same century, Paracelsus observed its analgesic effect on chickens and failed to follow up this discovery and apply it to humans. Michael Faraday noted in 1818 that ether produced an anesthesia similar to nitrous oxide. In 1842, William Clark, a medical student, gave ether to a patient undergoing a tooth extraction by Dr. Elijah Pope of Rochester, New York. This was the first extraction ever recorded using ether anesthesia. Crawford Long of Jefferson, Georgia, while a medical student at the University of Pennsylvania, along with other medical students, freaked-out with ether. The idea soon came to him to try ether for human surgery. In 1842, he excised a neck tumor under ether anesthesia. In 1849, Long reported his ether-anesthesia surgical cases in the *Southern Medical and Surgical Journal*.

William Morton of Massachusetts demonstrated the anesthetic property of ether at the Massachusetts General Hospital in 1846, by anesthetizing a patient for the eminent surgeon, John C. Warren, professor of surgery at Harvard. The procedure was published in the *Boston Medical and Surgical Journal* in 1846. Philadelphia physicians attacked this new method as quackery. However, the reputation of Warren gave its respectability, and ether anesthesia was adopted in Paris and London in the same year. Chloroform soon competed with ether. The foremost Scottish obstetrician, James Simpson, used ether and, in 1847, switched to chloroform, using it with excellent results in delivering many babies. While theologians denounced chloroform anesthesia as being contrary to the biblical teaching that "In sorrow shalt thou bring forth children," the method was widely adopted after Queen Victoria chose chloroform for anesthesia during the birth of her seventh child.

The use of anesthetics changed the course of surgery and allowed surgeons to take more time and do more complicated surgery than ever before possible. Up to this time, surgeons had to quickly rush through operations while groaning and screaming patients were forcibly restrained. The best surgeon was considered to be the quickest operator. Yet, despite this great discovery, surgical operations were accompanied with a high mortality. Simple operations had an attendant mortality of 30% and complicated surgery was accompanied by a very high death rate. In fact, most people feared surgery, and the hospital was considered a death house. Infection was a prime cause of such deaths, and we shall say more about this later.

The next great American physician was the poet-physician Oliver Wendell Holmes (1809-1894), professor of anatomy at Harvard.

He wrote an epochal work, the Contagiousness of Puerperal (childbirth) Fever in 1843, five years before the great Semmelweiss. He pointed out that physicians carried disease from one pregnant mother to another or from a contagious case to the expectant mother. He was also a great believer in the healing power of nature and a strong opponent of drug overdosing.

Austin Flint (1812-1866) was called the American Laennec because of his prolific use of the stethoscope. He wrote 200 articles and 6 books embracing diseases of the chest, auscultation and percussion, diseases of the heart, and principles and practice of medicine. A heart murmur was named after him. No man influenced medicine more than Austin Flint in his time.

Marion Sims (1813-1883) was the American father of Gynecology (women's diseases). This brilliant physician was the first surgeon to cure a bladder-vaginal fistula by surgery. Up to this time, women suffering from the leakage of urine into the vagina were doomed to a life of misery and agony. Sims' success made him world famous and he was invited to Europe to demonstrate his technique. Sims devised a new position for examining and operating on his patients, known ever since as the Sims' position, where the woman lies on her side. He also introduced, for his surgical procedure, a new kind of vaginal speculum, the so-called duck billed type, to observe the vagina and uterine opening "as no man had ever seen before." He used a silver wire suture to avoid infection, and a catheter to empty the bladder while the fistula between the bladder and vagina was healing.

Samuel Gross (1805-1884) was one of the most famous surgeons of his era. He was a prolific writer and among his works was the famous "System of Surgery" written in two volumes and consisting of 2360 pages, profusely illustrated.

Before we move into the stimulating and exciting second half of the nineteenth century there are two German surgeons who deserve mention. Carl von Graefe (1787-1840) was the founder of modern plastic surgery. He devised operations for cleft palate, rhinoplasty (nose rebuilding), and blepharoplasty (eyelid repairs). Johann Diffenbach (1792-1847) treated strabismus (cross-eyedness) by cutting eye muscles, performed skin grafting, and was a pioneer in animal transplantation of tissues.

The French School continued to enjoy success in the second half of the nineteenth century. One of their outstanding men was

Claude Bernard (1813-1878). He made several important discoveries in physiology. First, he showed that digestion was not solely a stomach function, but that the pancreatic juices contributed enzymes to digest fats, proteins and starches. Secondly, he discovered that sugar is stored in the liver as glycogen, and, when needed, glycogen is converted to sugar for immediate release. Thirdly, he discovered that there are two types of vasomotor nerves to blood vessels, one that constricts and the other that dilates. Among other contributions he made were: 1) an injury to the floor of the brain near the cerebellum produces a temporary diabetes in animals; 2) in carbon monoxide poisoning, carbon monoxide replaces oxygen in red blood cells; 3) the drug curare blocks nervous impulses at the junction between nerve and muscle thereby causing paralysis. Bernard never practiced medicine.

Brown-Sequard (1817-1894), of French-American background, was born on the British island of Mauritius. Among his contributions are the well-known Brown-Sequard syndrome, in which destruction of one half the spinal cord results in loss of sensation on the opposite side of the body and retention of sensation on the same side below the lesion or injury. Like Bernard, and unaware of his work, he reported that stimulation of the sympathetic nerves of the neck cause constriction of the blood vessels of the face, resulting in blanching or the face turning pale. He also proved the adrenals are necessary to life, and produced Addison's disease by their removal. He used extracts from testicles to try to rejuvenate old men, and believed, along with Claude Bernard, in the internal secretions theory. He felt that internal secretions were produced and secreted into the blood by the adrenals, liver, pancreas, spleen, kidneys, and sex glands, and that such substances could be utilized in treating disorders of these organs.

The Austrian school of Vienna came into prominence in the second half of this century by the remarkable work of three men—Rokitansky and Skoda, both Czechs, and Hebra, a Moravian. Carl Rokitansky (1804-1878) was the outstanding pathologist of his time, having performed with his assistants almost 60,000 regular autopsies and 25,000 medico-legal autopsies. He differentiated between lobar and bronchopneumonia, described and named acute yellow atrophy of the liver, and found bacteria on the valves of the heart in severe endocarditis. His contributions were voluminous. Joseph Skoda (1805-1881) was a specialist in percussion and auscultation, improvising new names for the various sounds. He was a therapeutic nihilist, one who believed that there was no available treatment for disease. He was considered one of the best diagnosticians and teachers of his age. His chief claim to fame is his famous textbook on percussion and auscultation. He opposed bleedings, emetics, and purgings for treating pneumonia and believed, correctly, that more patients would recover if left alone.

Ferdinand Hebra (1816-1880) was the first Viennese dermatologist. Little was known about skin diseases in his day, and they were treated with antimony and laxatives. Blood impurities were blamed for skin eruptions and ulcers. Hebra found, however, that such was not the case. He discovered that scabies was due to the itch mite and its death resulted in cure. Eczema could be produced by skin irritants and cleared with local treatment. He wrote a famous textbook on dermatology and considered most skin disorders as purely local in origin and needing local therapy. He revised the use of mercury in treating syphilis. Yet in the main, he, like Skoda, was a therapeutic nihilist, believing that most diseases got well by themselves.

Ignatz Semmelweiss (1815-1865), a Hungarian member of the Viennese school, observed that puerperal or childbirth fever was caused by the unclean, disease-carrying hands of the examining physicians. He ordered all physicians under his jurisdiction to wash their hands with calcium chloride before inserting them into their female patients. This was the first mandatory use of antisepsis. The death rate on his obstetrical service eventually fell to zero in 1848. Semmelweiss was bitterly attacked and persecuted by his fellow obstetricians for his ideas. Eventually he went mad and died.

The students of these Vienna giants, Rokitansky, Skoda, and Hebra continued to carry on the glory of the Vienna School. They created the specialties of ophthalmology (eye), otology (ear), and laryngology (throat). In the latter half of the nineteenth century, Vienna became the city of choice for Americans to study medicine instead of Paris. Vienna was the peer for excellent medical instruction.

The birth of the German school of medicine may be considered to have started with Johannes Muller (1815-1858), the greatest German physiologist of his era. In his *Handbook of Human Physiology* he disclosed many new and novel facts on nerve energies, color sensations produced by pressure on the retina of the eye, and voice and vocal cord function. In chemistry, he discovered glutin and chondrin. He was among the first to use the microscope and described the appearance of tumors microscopically. He believed that fever was a nervous reflex. He was a mystic and, in a sense, ascribed to Stahl's theory of vitalism, holding the view that the soul or anima was the prime movement of life. Muller conducted extensive investigations in biology and zoology.

Carl Ludwig (1816-1895) was one of the most unselfish men of any time. He did a great deal of research work and published many of his articles under the names of his pupils instead of his own. In 1865, his institute at Leipzig was the world's leading physiological institute and students from all over the world sought his teaching. A few of his many contributions to medicine were the invention of the kymograph (an instrument for recording muscle and arterial variations), the blood pump, and the Stromuhr (for measuring blood flow). He formulated theories on urine formation, the physiology of the heartbeat, and the effects of drugs and nerve stimulation on the heart and circulation. One of his pupils, Cloetta, discovered uric acid, leucin, taurin, and inosite.

John Liebig (1803-1873) discovered hippuric acid, chloral, and chloroform. Liebig studied uric acid, devised a way to estimate urea, and studied blood, bile, fats, and meat juices. He wrote the first book on organic chemistry in 1842 and demonstrated the relationship between organic chemistry and physiology and pathology. Liebig is considered the founder of agricultural chemistry, physiological chemistry and carbon compounds chemistry. He taught, in opposition to prevalent medical opinions, that animal heat was due to oxidation and combustion in the tissues. Liebig, in collaboration with Friedich Wohler, published one of the most famous historical papers in chemistry, that of benzaldhydes.

Wohler (1800-1882) in 1824, at the age of 24, made a monumental discovery in chemistry by showing that the ingestion of benzoic acid would result in hippuric acid being excreted in the urine, demonstrating that animals, like plants, can elaborate complex chemicals. Later it was found that uric acid could be synthesized from ammonium carbonate, and glycogen from glucose. Wohler in 1828 made another epochal discovery. He heated ammonium cyanate and produced urea, the first time an organic substance had been created from an inorganic compound without intervening life processes, thus demonstrating the close relationship between the chemistry of living and non-living substances. This was the final blow to destroying the vitalist theories which had strong advocates up to this point in history. It was beginning to be appreciated that life processes were chemical.

Theodore Schwann (1810-1882) one of Muller's students, published a treatise in 1839 on his discovery that all plants and animals are composed of cells of varying appearances. Another German by the name of Schleiden published a similar paper in 1838 on the cell makeup of plants. Their monumental discovery is now known as the Schleiden-Schwann cell theory. While others had noted the same facts, it was these two men who strongly imprinted their findings on medical, biologic, and botanic sciences. Schwann also showed that fermentation is caused by a living substance, yeast, and that fermentation could be stopped by sterilization which killed the organisms. He also isolated pepsin, which digests proteins in the stomach, and discovered that bile is necessary for digestion in the bowel.

Jacob Henle (1809-1885), a pupil of Muller, was considered one of the greatest anatomists and microscopists of all times. In 1840, he published a monograph on contagious diseases in which he emphasized that a living substance caused such illnesses. Under his microscope, he examined material from contagious patients and saw various bacteria, but did not know exactly what they did. He also published books on anatomy and pathology in which he described his many discoveries. Henle was also a fine teacher and illustrator.

One of the most remarkable proteges of Muller was Herman Helmholtz (1821-1894) a brilliant scientist and physician. He proclaimed the law of conservation of energy, measured the velocity of nerve impulses, invented the ophthalmoscope for viewing the interior of the eye, revived the theory of color vision proposed by Thomas Young, concluded that there are three primary colors—blue, green, and red, studied the ear and made important findings in acoustics. In physics, Helmholtz made important contributions to thermodynamics, hydrodynamics, and electrodynamics. He believed that chemical atoms are ultimately electric in structure. In medicine, he was mostly investigative, but did suggest that quinine sulphate might be helpful if applied in the nose of hay fever sufferers. Among the scientists working in Helmholtz's laboratories was

Hertz, who discovered the electric Hertzian waves known now as radio waves. The work of Helmholtz and that of Emil du Bois Reymond (1818-1896) of Berlin was an incentive to study muscle and nerve physiology. Du Bois Reymond stimulated muscle-nerve preparations by a special coil he invented to give faradic electrical discharges. His work in this field gained him renown as the founder of modern electrophysiology.

Another of Muller's outstanding pupils was Rudolph Virchow (1821-1902). He was the creator of modern pathology. In 1848, he published his monumental work *Cellularpathology,* in which he emphasized that every cell came from a previous cell and that pathological cells were derived from normal cells as the result of stimulation or irritation. These cellular changes result in organic disease. For all time, Virchow now destroyed the ancient theories of the humors and other nonscientific theories to explain disease.

Virchow was the first to identify leukocytosis (increased amounts of white cells in the blood) and, along with John Bennett in 1845, he discovered leukemia (malignant condition of the white cells). He also formulated the "doctrine of embolism." Virchow showed that the older theories of embolism (clot formation and traveling in a blood vessel) were wrong. It was formerly held that thrombosis (clot formation) and pyemia (the products of pus producing disease appearing in the blood) followed phlebitis (inflamed vein). Instead, Virchow demonstrated that in phlebitis the thrombus occurred first. In his autopsies, Virchow often noted emboli in the lungs and brain. Virchow made many discoveries in medicine and, in addition, was a renowned anthropologist, archeologist, and historian.

After Virchow, there were other German medical geniuses. Julius Cohnheim (1839-1884), Virchow's pupil, demonstrated that, in inflammation, white cells leave the blood through capillary walls and form pus cells and pus in the tissues. Cohnheim also successfully inoculated rabbits with tuberculosis. Carl Weigert (1854-1904) was the first to stain bacteria for microscopic examination, making them easier for identification. Felix-Hoppe-Seyler (1825-1895), a great physiological chemist, isolated the red blood cell's hemoglobin which carries oxygen. Albrecht Kossel (1853-1927) performed very important work on the chemistry of the cell and its nucleus. The German chemists were responsible for isolating most of the amino acids which make up proteins. Heinrich Quincke

(1842-1922) described Quincke's disease known also as angioneurotic edema, an allergic swelling of the skin or mucus membranes. He also introduced lumbar puncture for removing spinal fluid for medical diagnosis. The list of German advances in medicine is long and of necessity much must be omitted.

The British school of medicine advanced along with its colleagues on the continent. British science had already established its solidity in the personages of Davy, Faraday, Dalton, and Owen.

In 1859, Charles Robert Darwin published his now famous *On the Origin of the Species by Means of Natural Selection*. This monograph was based upon his five years voyage aboard the Beagle, a British ship, which took him on a long voyage to Atlantic islands, South America, and islands in the Pacific and Indian oceans.

Alfred Wallace, in 1858, arrived at the same theory. Both had read and were impressed by the work of the clergyman Malthus on population explosion. In the struggle for existence, Darwin believed favorable variations would survive and unfavorable ones perish. In this way, new species would arise. In support of the evidence for evolution, Darwin presented facts from paleontology, biology, comparative anatomy and embryology, and the presence of vestigial or rudimentary organs, which are no longer functional. Darwin's publication destroyed for all time the concept of fixed species proposed in the 18th century by Linnaeus, which held that all plants and animals were created originally as we see them today. It also wiped out the idea that the universe was constructed solely for man. For Galileo had shown that the earth was not the center of the universe, but rather a minor planet in a vast spacial sea.

The concept of evolution is ancient. The Greeks, as we have shown previously, believed in it. So did Bacon, Erasmus, Goethe, Lamarck and others. But Darwin had collected much evidence in support of the idea. The publication of the *Origin* brought down the condemnation of both Catholic and Protestant clergymen. However, Darwin was a peaceful man and refused to get into polemics, living out his life peacefully.

There are, however, flaws in Darwin's theory. He did not consider occasional mutations, changes produced by spontaneous and accidental variations, which geneticists claim may also originate new species. Many animal characteristics are not the result of survival. However, with due respect, Darwin thought natural selection was the main reason for evolution, but he conceded that other factors might also be operative. A specific characteristic is of value in survival only if essential to an animal's environment and not as the result of an accidental enemy.

Thomas Huxley (1825-1895), famous physician, naturalist, biologist and paleontologist, was the vociferous champion for Darwin. He had, however, pointed out to Darwin some of the weaknesses in the theory of natural selection, but he still firmly believed in evolutionary processes. Huxley felt that natural selection alone was not the answer. His own observations on animal and human freaks were prophetic of Mendel's coming discoveries in genetics and, for lack of a better explanation, Huxley called this phenomenon the "doctrine of transmutation."

Since the chemical structure of DNA (Deoxyribonucleic acid, the genetic material of inheritance), was elicited in 1953, geneticists have questioned Darwin's theory of mutations. The great biologist "supposed" that mutations were infrequent and harmful. Modern molecular biologists say that random errors occur in DNA reduplication in mammalian genes at the rate of about one new allele (a gene which determines characteristics such as shortness or tallness) in the population every two years. Most of these genetic changes are of no consequence and in no way effect function. Therefore, they conclude, gross mutations result from "genetic drift," not survival of the fittest.

James Paget (1814-1899) was a great surgeon and pathologist. When a young man, he noted and dissected out small white objects in muscles. Under the microscope he found them to be small worms. This proved to be the causative factor in trichinosis, a disease caused by eating uncooked pork in which these worms are present. Moses had forbidden Hebrews to eat pork 3,000 years ago, having observed trichinosis, but not knowing the exact cause. Paget's name has been attached to two diseases. Paget's disease of the bone is known as osteitis deformans, in which the bones are deformed due to a softening and hardening process. Paget's disease of the nipple, which is an eczema, denotes impending or actual cancer of the breast.

Joseph Lister (1827-1912) was England's greatest surgeon. As a young physician he discovered two muscles in the iris, one which constricted the pupil of the eye and the other that dilated it. He also described the involuntary muscles in the skin which, upon contracting, produce what is popularly known as "goose pimples." Lister, however, is best known for his discovery of antisepsis. In his surgical experience, he was impressed by the appalling mortality rate from hospital surgery. Infected wounds were so common, with the pouring out of pus, that surgeons of Lister's time and generations past called the suppuration "laudable pus." They believed, in their profound ignorance, that infection was necessary for the healing of wounds, and the presence of pus was a good sign!

Lister noted that fractures which did not break through the skin, and were called simple fractures, healed rapidly with no complications. On the contrary, fractures that broke through the skin, and were called compound fractures, were frequently accompanied by infection, gangrene, and death. Surgical wounds also became infected and frequently followed the same course of events.

Lister was impressed by the work of Pasteur, in which the Frenchman showed that it was the germs in the air which produced sepsis. Lister determined to try carbolic acid as an antiseptic agent, having noted its success in this capacity in the treatment of sewage in the town of Carlisle. In 1865, Lister used carbolic acid-soaked cloth in compound fractures with excellent results. His success in preventing infection in compound fractures and surgical wounds too, prompted him to publish a monograph in 1867 announcing this discovery. He later realized that ligatures of silk and catgut, which were used for sewing and tying in surgery, could also provide sepsis. Therefore, he sterilized his ligatures with carbolic acid. In 1870, Lister sprayed the operating room with carbolic acid to kill microbes before they fell into wounds. About 17 years later he abandoned the idea as not being necessary. He was not wrong in his original thought, for today in many modern operating rooms, the air is treated with ultraviolet radiation to kill air-borne infection.

His novel contribution of antisepsis met with the usual reaction one might expect from his colleagues. He came under strong attack, but on the continent of Europe his concept was enthusiastically accepted by his peers. Lister, in eventually learning of Semmelweiss' previous work, acknowledged his priority. Unlike Semmelweiss, who was persecuted until he finally went out of his mind and died, Lister was enthusiastically received and honored on the continent, and finally in Britain he received one award after another, ultimately becoming a peer of the realm.

Drugs, Demons, Doctors, and Disease

Due to Lister's important discovery of antisepsis, the operating room and the surgeon were no longer the unwilling instruments of the angel of death. The ability to prevent surgical infection and the conquest of pain in operations by the use of anesthesia, constitute two of the greatest discoveries in medical history and they were both made in the nineteenth century.

An equally dramatic event in this century was the rapid advance made in bacteriology at about the same time as antisepsis. The founding fathers were Louis Pasteur and Robert Koch, both giants in this contribution.

The concept that minute invisible creatures or animals could cause disease is quite old. The ancients believed in demons entering the body to produce disease. Marcus Varro, in the first century B.C., thought that living micro-organisms could produce disease by entering body openings. Fracastorius, in 1546, in his book *Contagion* practically spelled out for us the whole germ theory of disease, but unfortunately had no microscope to prove his hypothesis. In 1658, Kircher, while looking through the microscope, saw "worms" in the blood of bubonic plague victims and "small animals" in rotting meat. Leeuwanhoek, the discoverer of spermatozoa, recognized certain bacilli, protozoa, and cocci, according to sketches he presented to the Royal Society of his time. But he did not associate his findings with disease.

The earliest pioneer in bacteriology was Agostino Bassi (1773-1856) who, in 1835, showed that a living parasite infected silkworms and that this material, if applied to a healthy silkworm, reproduced the same disease. He showed how to prevent the disease by segregating the healthy worms, and treating the infected areas of silkworms with chemicals to eradicate the disorder.

Other investigators in the early years of the nineteenth century saw micro-organisms in various liquids such as water, wine, vinegar, blood, and milk. Henle, in 1840, suggested that infectious diseases were due to living agents. Pollender in 1849 and Davaine and Rayer in 1850 observed the anthrax bacillus in the blood of sheep which had succumbed to this disease.

Louis Pasteur's (1822-1895) discoveries were foremost in the bacteriological advances of the last century. He showed in 1857 that alcoholic fermentation of sugar was due to microscopic organisms and that lactic acid production, which soured milk, was due to another type of microorganism. He settled the controversy about spontaneous generation of life in solutions by demonstrating that microscopic organisms were not created spontaneously but were air contaminants. He showed that sterile infusion of material in a flask open to the air will putrefy, while if the neck of the flask is drawn out in curves and then to a very fine point, the material will not decompose; for the air-born germs cannot enter the infusion. In 1864, the wine industry of Jura was being ruined by parasitic growths which destroyed the wine. Pasteur recommended heating the wine for a few minutes to a temperature of between 50 to 60 degrees centigrade. This procedure killed the parasites and solved the problem. The heat process became known as "pasteurization," named after the master himself. Similar problems in the beer industry were successfully overcome by pasteurization, a method that is still applied today to milk and other perishables.

Next, between 1877 and 1881, Pasteur helped to conquer anthrax in sheep and cholera in chickens. Both diseases were decimating the respective animals in large numbers. Pasteur isolated the anthrax bacillus. He found that by heating a culture of these germs to 42 degrees centigrade he could reduce their virulence. Then, if they were used as a vaccine and injected into sheep, immunity to anthrax was produced. Pasteur isolated the chicken cholera organism in culture and discovered, accidentally, that when the culture got old the microbe lost its virulence. Then, when used as a vaccine, immunity was produced in chickens with no resulting harm.

Pasteur's most dramatic discovery came with the development of a vaccine from dried rabies-infected spinal cord. Dessication reduced the virulence of the rabies virus. In 1885, Pasteur treated a 9-year-old Alsatian boy bitten by a rabid dog with this rabies vaccine, and the boy lived. The bite of a rabid animal was always fatal. So stirred by this fantastic news was the world, that money poured into Paris from all over the globe to build an institution for Louis Pasteur to continue his researches. The drive was successful and the Pasteur Institute was dedicated in 1888, but unfortunately Pasteur was too ill to continue any further work. An international celebration was held in Paris on his 70th birthday in 1892. Pasteur died in 1895, having received all the honors France could bestow on her gallant son. We might mention two of his most famous sayings at this point: "In the fields of observation, chance favors only the prepared mind." "Science should not concern itself in any way with the philosophical consequences of its discoveries."

Drugs, Demons, Doctors, and Disease

While a devout Catholic, Pasteur believed that science and religion were both distinct, and, in the present stage of imperfect human knowledge, one should not allow them to "trespass on each other ....."

Robert Koch (1843-1910) was 21 years younger than Pasteur. Jacob Henle had been one of his teachers. Koch was the first to culture a pure growth of the anthrax bacillus, announcing the discovery in 1876. Pasteur was beginning his work on anthrax at this time and confirmed Koch's findings. In 1877, Koch reported his isolation of 6 different kinds of bacteria which caused wound infections. His outstanding discoveries put him in the forefront of medical scientists. In 1882, Koch again did the impossible, discovering the tubercle bacillus, the cause of tuberculosis. This was one of his most spectacular achievements. In 1883, he discovered the cholera vibrio, the agent that produced cholera.

In 1890, Koch discovered tuberculin, the toxin elaborated by the tuberculosis germ. He felt it could be used as a vaccine to immunize people against tuberculosis. In this respect it failed, but it has been useful ever since in skin testing to determine past or present tuberculous infection.

Koch was one of the greatest bacteriologists of all time. With thorough German precision he did what no other man had done previously, he produced pure cultures of the organisms he had isolated, so that he could reproduce the disease and study its pathology. Until his time, only two germs had been discovered as causative factors for two diseases, namely anthrax and relapsing fever. Koch provided the stimulating impetus to further microbic research.

Rapidly, after Koch, the microbe agents responsible for many diseases were isolated:

ISOLATOR	MICROBE	DISEASE
Hansen (1871-74)	lepra bacillus	leprosy
Neisser (1879)	gonococcus	gonorrhea
Eberth (1880)	typhoid bacillus	typhoid fever
Frankel (1884)	pneumococcus	pneumonia
Kleks (1883)	diptheria bacillus	diptheria
Loeffler (1883-84)		
Nicolaier (1884)	tetanus bacillus	tetanus
Weishselbaum (1887)	meningococcus	meningitis
Kitasato (1894)	plague bacillus	bubonic plague
Bordet		

95

Drugs, Demons, Doctors, and Disease

ISOLATOR	MICROBE	DISEASE
Gengou (1906)	Bordet-Gengou bacillus	whooping cough
Pasteur (1878-79)	strepticoccus pyogenes	boils, puerperal
	staphylococcus pyogenes	infection, wound infections
Escheric (1886)	colon bacillus	peritonitis, intestional infections, skin infection
Bruce (1887)	brucella	Malta fever
Shiga (1897)	Shiga's bacillus	dysentery
van Emergem	botulinus bacillus	food poisoning

In the field of parasitology, many important discoveries were also made.

Leidy (1840) on trichina spiralis (trichinosis—pork worm)
Lasch (1875) on ameba (amebic dysentery)
Kuchenmeister (1853) on tapeworm infestations
vonSeibold (1854) on taenia (a type of tapeworm) and hydatids (a tapeworm known as cysticerus)
Scholein (1839) on favus (a fungus)
Muller (1841) on psospermosis (a protozoa)
Dubini (1843) on anchylostomiasis (hookworm)
Laveran (1880) on malaria parasites
Bennett (1842) on the aspergillosis fungus
von Langenback (1848) on the ray fungus also known as actinomycosis
Nocard (1880) on the nocardiosis fungus
Schenck (1898) on the sporotrichosis fungus

How are some of these strange diseases transmitted to humans? The ancients believed in demon infiltration of the body. Eventually other ideas were considered. For example, in the Sanskrit Susruta it was believed that the mosquito could transmit malaria. Nott (1848) and Beauperthuy (1854) also held the same idea. Laveran (1880) saw parasites in the blood of the malaria patients. Grassi and Bignami in 1899 showed that malaria parasites could only develop in the Anopheles mosquito and Ross (1898) demonstrated the parasites in the salivary glands of the same mosquito. Manson (1900) showed that malaria was definitely transmitted by the bite of the infected mosquito, as did Grassi and Bignami in malarial infested country. Manson, however, had malarial infected mosquitoes sent to him from Italy and allowed them to bite his own son, who came down shortly with malaria. The clinching evidence here was that biting took place in a non-malarial region. It was now clear that drainage of swamps which gave sanctuary to the anopheles mosquito would wipe out the mosquito population and hence malaria. Manson, in 1879 while in China, demonstrated that filariasis Bancrofti, a disease due to a threadlike worm, may produce a massive enlargement of the male scrotum and legs. This condition is also called elephantiasis and was transmitted by infected mosquitoes.

The ancients believed that swampy regions caused malaria and the Romans drained the marshes to get relief from the disease. The name malaria itself was coined by Francesco Torti who wrote a treatise on malarial fevers in 1712 and devised the name "malaria" from "mal" and "aria" meaning bad air. Modern research disclosed 4 types of parasites which cause human malaria. They give rise to chills, fevers, and sweating. Attacks occur daily, on alternate days or every two days, depending on the parasite causing the disorder. The uninfected mosquito bites a human infected with the parasites, absorbs them from the blood and then later transmits the disease by biting a human.

If flies could zoom through the air, and demons could assuredly do so, then possibly flies could also transmit disease. Perhaps in a way they were demons. The ancients had an intuitive feeling that flies may have had some relationship to pestilences.

The Egyptians wore fly and flea amulets to ward off disease. The Babylonian god, Nergal, was lord of pestilence and appeared in the form of an insect. In the Bible there is recorded a plague of flies which smote the Egyptians. Beelzebub, Lord of the flies, was a Philistine deity with the power to send or remove plagues of flies. He is referred to in the Bible.

More discerning observations on flies have been made by physicians. Ambrose Pare' in 1557 noted that flies were disease carriers at the battle of St. Quentin. Leidy in 1865, during the Civil War, also noted this fact in his own hospital. Raimbert, in 1869, showed that flies transmit anthrax, Tizzoni and Cattani in 1886 felt that cholera was being carried by these insects. Grassi observed that eggs of intestinal worms were being transported by flies, and Celli noted that flies cárry tuberculosis and typhoid germs. Others have shown that Kala-azar and trypanosomiasis were also spread by these vectors.

An epidemic of yellow fever broke out in Havana, Cuba, in 1900 and a commission of Walter Reed, James Caroll, Jesse Lazear, and Aristides Agramonte was sent by the U. S. army to study the disease. They worked closely with J. C. Gorgas, the sanitary engineer of Havana, and Carlos Finlay who insisted the disease was transmitted by mosquitoes. His idea was treated with much scepticism. Eventually, he was vindicated and the mosquito, now known as the aedes aegypti, was proven to be the culprit. Gorgas wiped out yellow fever in Havana in three months by eradicating the mosquito. Then 4 years later, he freed the Panama Canal Zone from mosquitoes thus enabling the USA to build the canal, where the French had failed due to yellow fever and malaria.

As an interesting commentary we may mention the following. Recently, ancient human feces were found in caves in western Utah. They were dated at 9500 B.C. and 7837 B.C. One showed the presence of a thorny-headed worm, the other a pinworm. How long has man been invaded by worms? Probably as long as man and worm have existed side by side.

In the nineteenth century, many new drugs were introduced. A list of the important ones appears below. Most were new, others restudied and new uses found.

YEAR	INTRODUCER	NAME OF DRUG	USE
1805	Seturner	Morphine	narcotic
1817	Pelletier	Emetine	dysentery
1818	Thenard	Hydrogen Peroxide	oxidant
1818	Caventou & Pelletier	Strychinine	stimulant
1819	Caventou & Pelletier	Brucine	a bitter
1820	Caventou & Pelletier	Veratrine	slows pulse
1820	Caventou & Pelletier	Quinine	malaria
1820	Dumas	Iodine	goitre
1822	Serul	Iodoform	antiseptic
1822	Scherer	Cod Liver Oil	tonic
1827	Reichenbach	Creosote	antiseptic
1831	Blaud	Blaud's Pills (ferric carbonate)	anemia
1831	Guthrie Liebig Soubeiran	Chloroform	anesthetic
1832	Robiquet	Codeine	narcotic
1842	Long	Ether	anesthetic
1846	Morton	Ether	anesthetic
1846	Gobley	Lecithin	food supplement
1856	Jobst & Hesse	Physostigmin	smooth muscle stimulant

Drugs, Demons, Doctors, and Disease

YEAR	INTRODUCER	NAME OF DRUG	USE
1864	Hlasivetz Barth	Resorcin	antiseptic
1867	Brunton	Amyl Nitrate	angina pectoris
1869	Liebreich	Chloral	hypnotic
1873	Hardy Gerard	Pilocarpin	diaphoretic
1875	Chesebrough	Vaseline	lubricant
1876	Kolbe	Salicylic Acid	antipyretic
1882	Biebrichs	Scarlet Red	antiseptic
1884	Anrep	Cocaine	local anesthetic
1885	von Jaksch	Urethane	sleep producer
1885	Fraser	Strophanthus	heart tonic
1886	Unna	Ichthyol	skin disorders
		Resorcin	skin disorders
1886	von Nencki	Salol	bowel antiseptic
1886	Kahn & Hepp	Acetanilide	antipyretic
1887	Kast & Hinsberg	Phenacetine	antipyretic.
1887	Nagai	Ephedrine	asthma
1891	Giesel	Tropococaine	anesthetic
1893	Filehne & Spiro	Pyramidon	antipyretic
1894	Nicolaier	Urotropin	urinary antiseptic
1894	Oliver & Schafer	Suprarenal Extract	hormones
1894	von Behring	Diptheria Antitoxin	diptheria
1895	Calmette	Antiserum	venomous snake bites
1896	Merling	Eucaine	local anesthetic
1898	Dresser	Heroin	narcotic
1899	Gautier	Sodium Cacodylate	alterative
1899	Loeffler	Vaccine	hoof and mouth disease
1899	Dreser	Aspirin	antipyretic

A most interesting man of this century was Elia Metchnikoff (1845-1916), who discovered the principle of phagocytosis or devouring cells. Metchnikoff noted that when foreign substances or bacteria entered a living animal, its body would react by sending certain cells, called phagocytes, to engulf and destroy the invader. He studied the inflammatory reaction produced in this process, and concluded that immunity to infectious diseases was solely the action of these destroying cells. He later demonstrated that phagocytes originate at certain sites in the body called the reticuloendothelial system, which is located in the liver, bone marrow, lymph nodes, and spleen.

Metchnikoff wrote books on inflammation, immunity, and on

The Nature of Man. In the latter, he emphasized the serious effects of intestinal "auto-intoxication" and felt that the ingestion of lactic acid-producing bacteria would counteract the poisons of ordinary bacteria living in the intestine, and thereby prolong life. He advocated, therefore, the eating of yoghurt or curdled milk because he believed that Bulgarian peasants enjoyed a supposed longevity because of this food consumption, a conjecture later found not to be true.

An interesting and important discovery of the nineteenth century was that of the hypodermic syringe. Primitive Indians antedated this instrument with the use of a turkey quill to which an animal bladder was attached. Through this contrivance they forced water into the rectum for enema purposes. This device may be considered a primitive syringe. Hero of Alexandria, an inventive Greek genius of the first century A.D., was reported to have made and used a crude syringe of metal. Over the succeeding centuries, hypodermic instruments of various types were utilized. Not too much is known about them. After Harvey discovered the circulation of the blood, the blood vessels of cadavers (corpses) were injected with colored materials, using crude syringes, so that they could be seen and studied better. DeGraaf invented a new syringe in 1668 and used it to inject spermatic vessels.

Rynd in 1845 introduced the gravity-type syringe which he had invented. A pressure-type hypodermic syringe was employed by Provaz in 1851 and Wood in 1855. Barker in 1856 and Elliott in 1858 were the first Americans to employ this new syringe. These instruments were metal. In the twentieth century, the glass syringe superceded the metal one, only to be replaced later by the plastic disposable device. Special tablets, which could be dissolved and used for hypodermic injection, were invented and introduced by Robert Fuller of Philadelphia in 1878.

Intravenous injection of drugs, which was first recorded in the 17th century, and then abandoned, was revived by Gaspard and Magendie in 1823 in order to study the reaction of drugs given in this fashion.

G. B. Halford in 1869 reintroduced the treatment of snake bites with ammonia, first advocated by Fontana in 1767. However, Halford injected the ammonia hypodermically, instead of applying it locally like Fontana. Guido Bacelli gave injections of quinine for malaria in 1890 and mercury for syphilis in 1894. In 1887, Pitres

Drugs, Demons, Doctors, and Disease

and Vaillard suggested the injection of alcohol into nerves for painful neuralgia to stop the discomfort, but they never performed the procedure. Schloesser in 1903 was the first to institute this therapy.

Carlo Forlaini in 1895 injected air into the chest, which is called artificial pneumothorax, to treat tuberculosis of the lung, a suggestion made in 1842 by Carson. This technique was introduced into America by James Murphy in 1898. The air injection collapses the lung, thereby allowing it to rest and heal.

Many studies and advances were made in the field of dietetics. William Banting initiated the treatment of obesity in 1863 with a diet restricting fats and carbohydrates. Ewald and Boas used special test meals in diagnosing stomach disorders. Von Norden studied metabolic disorders and concluded that an oatmeal diet would benefit diabetics. Outstanding investigators during this century were Beaumont, Chittenden, Iiebig, Pavloff, and Wohler. Jukes and Bush, in 1822, introduced the stomach pump for removing poisons from the stomach, whether taken accidentally or deliberately.

Silas Weir Mitchell (1829-1914) was the outstanding neurologist of his time. This Philadelphian made many new discoveries in his specialty. Among these were the disorder of ascending neuritis, the psychology of amputations, and reflex paralysis. He is best known, though, for the "Weir Mitchell Treatment," also known as the "Rest Treatment," which he introduced in 1879. Mitchell advocated treating nervous disorders by a combination of prolonged rest in bed, a good diet, massage, and electric therapy. Mitchell's treatment was quickly employed throughout the world and he soon acquired an international reputation.

One of the most spectacular discoveries in physics and medicine was made by William Conrad Rontgen on November 8, 1895. This physicist, while passing an electric current through a Crookes tube covered with black paper, noted a fluorescence occuring in some barium platinocyanide crystals lying on the table. Intrigued by this phenomenon, Rontgen made a screen of the same material which also glowed when exposed to the emanations from the current-activated tube. When he placed his hand between the tube and screen he saw the outline of his hand bones on the screen. Then he replaced the screen with a photographic plate and obtained a permanent record of the event. In December 1895, Rontgen published his results and, not knowing what the rays were, called them x rays.

The medical uses of this facinating discovery were quickly forthcoming. In the Graeco-Turkish War of 1897 and the Spanish American War of 1898, x rays were used to diagnose bone fractures and to disclose the location of bullets. In 1899, Stenbech treated cancer with these rays. The use of x rays to probe into the gastrointestinal, genito-urinary, and other systems of the human body soon followed. One of the most important physical tools for diagnosis had been found. In 1898, the Curies announced their discovery of radium. This radiation was also quickly applied to cancer treatment.

American medicine was coming of age in the nineteenth century. William Osler (1849-1920) was probably the most famous physician of his time and made the greatest impact upon American medicine. He advocated, for American students, the excellent medical training that German universities offered. He himself trained at McGill University in Canada, then went to Europe to advance his medical knowledge. Osler was appointed physician-in-chief at the new Johns Hopkins Hospital and professor of medicine at the Johns Hopkins University in 1877. Together with William Welch, pathologist, Howard Kelly, gynecologist, and William Halsted, surgeon, he formed the nucleus of the famous Johns Hopkins Medical School which opened in 1893.

Osler resolved to build a great medical institution along Germanic lines. Before a student could be admitted, he had to have a reading knowledge of either German or French and be a college graduate. He must have also completed courses in biology, physics, and chemistry. These extraordinary requirements stirred the American medical profession, which had a rather low educational standard. The Johns Hopkins Medical School raised the standard of medical education in America. In addition it also established the first system of residencies in medicine, surgery, obstetrics and gynecology.

Osler wrote one of the most famous American medical texts, *The Principles and Practice of Medicine*. This book was translated into many foreign languages. Osler was a man of extreme charm, an inspiring teacher, an outstanding speaker and witty writer. His book was called to the attention of John D. Rockefeller, who was deeply inspired, and as a result the millionaire founded the Rockefeller Institute for Medical Research.

Osler made no profound discovery. He was an early investigator of blood platelets in 1873, discovered in 1877 the filiaria which caused bronchitis in dogs, observed polycythemia rubra (excessive red cells in the blood which give a ruddy complexion) in 1903, and described red swellings, known as Osler's spots, in severe endocarditis of the heart. Osler was a great medical historian and was also the editor of several outstanding medical journals. Garrison called him "the greatest physician of our time."

Welch (1850-1934) was also a dynamic person, being an excellent lecturer and teacher. He was the first dean of The Johns Hopkins medical school. Welch was responsible for developing a group of outstanding pathologists, raising pathology to a fitting high-status in America. He discovered the Welch bacillus, known as aerogenes capsulatus which causes gas gangrene, and also the staphylococcus epidermidis albus in 1892. He described changes produced in the body by injections of diptheria toxin.

William Halsted (1852-1922) was an austere type of person, unlike Welch and Osler. He was one of America's most capable surgeons. In 1884 he saved the life of a patient suffering from carbon monoxide poisoning by reinfusing aerated blood. In 1885, he introduced a new type of drain for wounds called the "cigarette drain." He invented rubber gloves for surgery in 1890 and described anesthesia with cocaine for regional anesthesia.

Howard Kelly (1858-1943) was an early user of local anesthesia and also invented new instruments and procedures. Among his instruments were the Kelly clamp to stop bleeding and the rectoscope for rectal examinations.

Reginald Fitz (1843-1913) in 1879 became professor of pathology at Harvard. In 1866, he stated that appendicitis was a cause of disease and death. This discovery is credited as being among the important advances in medicine of the 19th century. In the same year in which he made this announcement, Kronlein of Zurich surgically removed the appendix, a procedure known as appendectomy, in a patient suffering from acute appendicitis.

The nineteenth century saw many impressive achievements in medicine. The introduction of auscultation and x rays made diagnosis more possible and precise. Medicine moved into the scientific sphere when Virchow destroyed once and for all the ancient theory of the four humors as being the cause of disease and substituted his cellular disease theory. Microscopic improvement and refinements helped Virchow and other investigators to see the actual disease processes taking place in tissues.

Bacteriology moved rapidly ahead and the infectious agents causing many diseases were discovered. The mythological demons of disease turned out to be microbiotic organisms. Antisepsis, aspetic surgery, and anesthesia made surgery a much safer procedure. The introduction of newer methods to prevent, control, and cure disease, which had plagued mankind for thousands and perhaps millions of years and which killed unknown billions of humans, were the highlights of the century.

A needed revolution in nursing care took place in this era due to the heroic efforts of Florence Nightingale (1820-1910), who was horrified by the atrocious nursing care given in English hospitals. She determined to devote her life to rectifying this situation. She went abroad to Germany and France to study the latest methods of nursing and then returned to England to further advance her knowledge. Due to her proficiency, she was chosen to head a woman's hospital in London in 1853.

In 1854, news of the sufferings of the British Army in the Crimean War reached London. Miss Nightingale was frightened by the disturbing news and took a group of nurses to the war zone with her to give all possible help. She was appalled by what she saw in the hospital at Scutari. It was a scene of filth, primitive sanitation, vermin, and a fantastically high death rate. Due to heroic work of the understaffed nurses, Miss Nightingale was able to markedly reduce the death rate and bring nursing order out of almost complete chaos. As a result, she became a national heroine, was highly honored, and with public help she opened a splendid school for nurses at St. Thomas' Hospital which became the model for all future schools of nursing in both Britain and the United States. Modern nursing recognizes Florence Nightingale as its founder and guiding light.

In 1859, J. Henri Dunant, while traveling through northern Italy, happened to observe the bloody battle of Soliferino between the Austrians and the combined troops of Italy and France. Three hundred thousand men were engaged and forty thousand casualties resulted. Dunant was appalled by the horror and lack of care for the wounded and dying. As a result of this terrible experience he organized the Red Cross. Yet few have ever heard of this man or know of his trials in trying to get nations to agree to cooperate and respect the principles in the code of ethics of the Red Cross. Dunant spent his fortune in doing this work and died a poor and practically forgotten man.

In concluding our impressions of the nineteenth century, we must emphasize certain facts with reference to medical care. Most physicians were poorly trained; The Johns Hopkins Medical School graduates and those graduating from a few other schools were the exception. The average doctor's equipment usually consisted of a thermometer and stethoscope. He did not possess electrical instruments for examination of the eye or ear, nor did he possess a flashlight. Similarly, there were no instruments for getting the blood pressure, no electrocardiograms, no basal metabolism testings, and no blood chemistry evaluations. The doctor did not have tests for syphilis or typhoid fever, blood cultures and sputum examinations for tuberculosis were not performed. He could, however, test urine for albumin and sugar.

The average doctor could not do very much for his patients, because medicine at the turn of the century was primitive, and what was known was of little help to the physician who did not possess the facilities to utilize it. Scurvy and beri-beri were the only two recognized deficiency diseases, the first being due to lack of vitamin C and the latter to a lack of vitamin B. Smallpox and rabies were the two diseases for which there were vaccines. The only antitoxin known was for diphtheria. While the physician recognized the contagiousness of smallpox, polio, measles, mumps, chickenpox, influenza, and German measles there was nothing he could do about them. No bacteria could be cultivated from these patients and so it was believed that the cause was some submicroscopic organism, also called a virus or poison.

There was no prenatal care for pregnant women. The first time most of them saw the doctor was when they were in labor. There was little to offer for complications and many died.

Tuberculosis was diagnosed by symptoms, history, and the physical findings. There was no treatment available and often many members of one family contracted the disease and died.

Transfusions of blood, intravenous infusions of saline, glucose, or minerals were unknown. No antibiotics were yet available, nor was insulin or antidiabetic drugs. The cause of syphilis was unknown and treatment consisted of taking potassium iodide orally and rubbing mercury ointment into the skin. A cliche of that day stated that "one night with Venus, meant three years with Mercury." There was no treatment of value in gonorrhea, although injections were given into the urethra. Barbiturates and tranquilizers were unknown. Opium was used by the laity for pain and insomnia.

A few drugs were generally available for treatment such as quinine for malaria, tincture of iodine and alcohol for skin disinfection, boric acid and zinc sulfate for eye disorders, digitalis for cardiac conditions. Local anesthetics such as novocaine were unknown. Ether, chloroform, and cocaine were available. Hormones of the adrenal, thyroid, and pituitary glands were not yet discovered.

Pneumonia was the big and dreaded killer. No effective treatment was known. All sorts of remedies were used, some definitely harmful, Pneumonia was known as the "Captain of the Men of Death." Lobar pneumonia killed one out of four healthy young people, in the elderly it was mostly fatal.

Due to unsanitary conditions, babies died very frequently of what was called dysentery or cholera infantum. This epidemic was most prevalent in the summer. Raw unpasteurized milk, which became contaminated with bacterial overgrowth in the summer time, killed thousands of infants. Contaminated foods contributed also to this decimation of children.

Another great killer of the populace was typhoid fever. Animal manure and human excreta littered the countryside contributing to pollution of water supplies. Typhoid carriers were not recognized, so as a result springs and wells became disseminators for typhoid germs, resulting in periodic typhoid epidemics. Typhoid carriers who handled food also spread the disease.

What the old time physician had was the drug morphine to allay pain, and a sense of dedication. He supplied moral support and his patients had great faith in him. He supplied the will to live and gave encouragement. Many times this made the difference between survival and non-survival.

Chapter Six

THE TWENTIETH CENTURY

THE TWENTIETH CENTURY began with high expectations that mankind would remain at peace, medical advancements would completely conquer disease, and that life would reach a glorious plane of social existence. Seven decades later these utopian and ideal aspirations of mankind still remain an unfulfilled dream.

Fielding Garrison, the great medical historian of a half-century ago, believed that the essential goal of medicine was preventive. It is ironic and sad to read of his predictions for the future, for he undoubtedly had high hopes fifty years ago. How far short we have come in these five decades the reader can easily decide. Garrison believed we would attain purification of water, air, soil, foods, and sewage; achieve complete hygienic methods for home and factory; improve and eventually eliminate slums; acquire good city planning; control alcoholism and drug addiction; control and eliminate venereal disease, tuberculosis, and cancer; adopt a sane, realistic, scientific attitude towards sex, replacing the anachronistic shackles of Victorian hypocrisy.

Instead of peace, mankind has plunged into a series of wars, the like of which has never been witnessed on this planet. Whether man will annihilate himself and his planet is yet to be seen. The peace that has been sought never came. Instead of purification we have massive pollution. The slums are still with us. Alcoholism and drug addiction have become worse. Venereal disease has grown more rampant due to sexual permissiveness, while tuberculosis has been more effectively treated and cancer is still a serious disease, although present methods of treatment and research may eventually control this dread affliction.

Yet, much has been accomplished in medicine in the last seven decades. Let us raise the curtain on the great advance made in this century, the greatest ever in the history of man. We have built well on the important discoveries of the nineteenth century. In view of the many advances, it is impossible to list all medical contributors and their discoveries. Only the most important will be described.

The discovery of adrenalin is one of the most interesting. It had been known that removal of the adrenal glands would result in death. In 1894, Oliver and Schafer discovered that a watery extract of these glands, when injected into the blood stream, produced a rise in blood pressure. In 1898, Abel isolated adrenalin, the first separation of a hormone in medical history. Takamine, in 1901, crystallized out the active principle itself, thus making it available in pure form. In 1904, Stolz synthesized adrenalin. Starling, in 1905, coined the term "hormone," meaning a chemical messenger, to describe internal secretions in the body.

Adrenalin is a natural drug. It is a powerful stimulant and increases blood pressure, heart contractions, heart rate, and heart output. It mimics in its action the sympathetic nervous system of the body. Adrenalin is used to resuscitate a heart which has stopped beating. It opens the tightly-constricting bronchial tubes in asthmatic attacks. Adrenalin is of value in heart and respiratory failure and has saved innumerable lives. It prolongs the action time of locally injected anesthetics. It can only be given by injection, for the digestive juices inactivate it. Side effects of the drug are tremors, nervous apprehension, palpitation, and distress in the region of the heart, known as precordial distress.

In 1901, Karl Landsteiner (1868-1943) discovered the various blood groups—O, A, B, and AB. Accordingly, it now became possible to cross-match blood before transfusions, thus avoiding transfusion reactions and possible deaths. In 1940, with Alexander Weiner, he found the Rh factor, important in obstetrics.

In 1903, Clemens von Pirquet and Bela Schick (discoverer of the Schick test for diphtheria) noted that the injection of diphtheria antitoxin, in a patient suffering from diphtheria, frequently produced what they called serum sickness. This occurred in about a week or ten days after the horse-serum antitoxin was injected. The patient might develop hives, asthma, joint swelling, and lymph node enlargement (swollen glands) or even die. Von Pirquet invented the name "allergy" to cover this phenomenon, meaning by it that there was an altered response in the body to the invasion of a foreign substance.

In the same year, Einthoven (1860-1927) created a remarkable instrument—the electrocardiograph. Since that time, physicians have been able to record electrical activity in the hearts of their patients. Such recordings are known as electrocardiograms and furnish valuable clues for diagnosing cardiac conditions.

In 1905, Fritz Schaudin (1871-1906) made a monumental discovery in medicine. For years, the cause of syphilis had evaded many investigators, but now Schaudin found the culprit. It was a corkscrew-looking microbe, which has been called by two different names—treponema pallidum or spirochaeta pallida. In 1906, a reliable test, the Wasserman test, was introduced for the diagnosis of syphilis from blood samples. In 1910, Paul Erlich (1854-1915), the father of modern chemotherapy finally found an effective treatment after 605 trials for this dread disease. He called it 606, for it was the 606th attempt. The drug was an arsenical preparation known as salvarsan, a powerful drug which often produced serious side reactions. It was only administered by intravenous injection.

A new form of salvarsan was eventually discovered which had less serious side reactions and was known as neosalvarsan. Along with this intravenous injection, mercury or bismuth compounds were injected into the buttocks. Thus the physician had a double barreled attack against syphilis. However, these were all powerful drugs and severe toxicity reactions could occur from their use. The effectiveness of penicillin in the 1940's obsoleted these drugs, and penicillin became the prime medication for treating syphilis. If there is an allergy to penicillin other antibiotics may be used.

In the last century, it had been demonstrated experimentally in animals that removal of the parathyroid glands, which are in close proximity to the thyroid gland and hence the name, resulted in convulsive seizures known as tetany, a condition which could end fatally. If such animals had parathyroid tissue transplanted, they would survive and the condition would not recur. The parathyroid glands control calcium levels in the blood, and, when removed the calcium content declines and tetanic spasms follow. Intravenous injection of calcium will quickly stop the convulsions. Vassale, in 1905, was the first to use parathyroid extract in treating tetany, and in 1925 Collip isolated the hormone of the parathyroids which was named parathormone.

In 1905, Einhorn discovered novocaine (procaine hydrochloride), a drug which is well known by the laity today. Until this time, physicians could only produce spinal or local anesthesia by the use of cocaine which is a dangerous and toxic drug. Novocaine is a much safer preparation and is still used today. In this same year of 1905 the Wright brothers flew the first heavier-than-air plane.

The pituitary gland was so named by Vesalius in the sixteenth century, because he believed (like Galen of the second century) that it received from the brain a phlegm or pituita, which it then secreted into the nose and pharynx to supply mucus. In 1894, Oliver and Schafer showed that injections of the pituitary raised blood pressure. In 1896, Howell demonstrated that such effects could only be achieved by extracts which came from the posterior or rear portion of the gland. In 1906, Dale noted that these extracts also caused the uterus to contract. Blair Bell used such extracts for sluggish labor in women from 1906 on. This uterine action of the drug is known as an oxytoxic response. Today either the natural extract of the pituitary or synthetics are utilized in inducing labor in women or for speeding up a lax, slow labor. Side effects are rare. These drugs should be carefully evaluated in abnormal labor. In overdoses, the drug may cause severe spasms and even rupture of the uterus. It also forces milk to pour out of nursing breasts, because it contracts the muscles in the milk ducts.

In 1911, Frank discovered that there was another hormone in the posterior pituitary which has an anti-diuretic effect. In the disease called diabetes insipidus (in contrast to diabetes mellitus or sugar diabetes), the patient passes enormous quantities of urine due to poor reabsorption of water by the kidney. The discovery of the second hormone in the pituitary, which combats diabetes insipidus, proves that the disease is due to inefficient manufacture of this hormone by the pituitary. In 1928, Kamm separated the two fractions of the gland and Vigneaud in 1953 isolated, identified and synthesized both the oxytoxic principle now called Pitocin, which also raises blood pressure, and the antidiuretic portion called Pitressin.

Between 1912-16, McCollum, Kennedy, and Davis discovered fat-soluble vitamin A, and water-soluble vitamin B, thus ushering in the age of vitamins.

Lack of vitamin A causes disorders of the surface-covering (epithelial) cells of the body, such as the skin and mucus membranes of the nose and respiratory tract, making them susceptible to disease and infection. The eyes are also adversely affected by a deficiency of vitamin A, which produces eye damage such as xerophthalmia or dry eye, night blindness, and keratomalacia or softening of the eyeball which may result in permanent blindness. Bone growth is also retarded.

This vitamin is present in yellow vegetables, butter and eggs. It is stored mostly in the liver and for this reason the liver, especially in fish, is one of the richest known sources of the vitamin. The ancient Egyptians administered fish oils to cure night blindness, never knowing why they worked. An intake of 5000 international units a day of vitamin A is considered essential. Overdosing of vitamin A can produce toxicity. Symptoms include fatigue, insomnia, bone and joint pain, loss of hair, peeling of the skin and pigmentation. Arctic explorers and Eskimoes have been poisoned by eating polar bear liver, due to the fact that this animal's liver is extremely high in vitamin A content. Acute intoxication follows such ingestion and the symptoms are nausea, vomiting, pain in the abdomen, headaches, and sleepiness—even death.

Lack of vitamin B is followed by beriberi, in which there may be widespread neuritis. It was eventually shown that vitamin B was made up of many different factors and that vitamin B_1 or thiamin was the essential component to prevent beriberi. The whole vitamin B complex is found in brewer's yeast, dried yeast and liver. Vitamin B_1 is found in cereal grains and other seeds, egg yolks and pork. About 1 mg per day is supposed to meet human needs. In 1926, Jansen and Donath isolated thiamin. This vitamin aids in the function of certain enzyme systems in which carbohydrates are converted into energy.

Thiamin is used to treat beriberi, gastrointestinal disturbances, alcoholic neuritis, disturbances of vision, pregnancy, pellagra, some types of anemia, and poor growth in children. It promotes a feeling of well-being and is utilized in many diseases and conditions for this purpose. Deficiency of this vitamin results in inflamation about the mouth (cheilosis) and tongue (glossitis), loss of weight, eye disturbances from light (photophobia), and skin disorders.

Vitamin B_2 or riboflavin is found in yeast, liver, organs and muscles of animals, some vegetables, and whole grains. It was recognized as a vitamin in 1933 by Kuhn, Gyorgy, and Wagner-Jauregg. About 2 mg is needed per day.

Nicotinic acid (niacin) deficiency produces pellagra. Goldberger demonstrated a missing dietary factor in 1925 and in 1937 Elvehjem and his associates identified the substance as nicotinic acid. In this disease, there is a redness of the skin on areas exposed to sunlight such as the hands, face, and neck. There is weakness and digestive disturbances, spinal pains, and in advanced cases, convulsons, mental disturbances, emaciation, and finally death. This disorder is seen in people who are mainly existing on corn. The vitamin is present, like other B factors mentioned, in yeast, liver, organs and muscles, and cereal grains. About 5 to 15 mg are required daily.

Nicotinic acid is used to treat pellagra, skin, gastrointestinal, and nervous system disorders and some types of anemia. It is also employed to lower blood cholesterol levels. Another utilization is to dilate blood vessels, especially in the lower extremities in some circulatory disorders.

Other vitamin B factors are employed in medicine. Vitamin B_{12} is given in pernicious anemia, other anemias, and sprue. In 1927, Minot and Murphy found that liver, in large amounts, would benefit pernicious anemia sufferers. Finally, in 1948, vitamin B_{12} was isolated in England and the USA When given by injection it brings pernicious anemia rapidly under control. B_{12} is often utilized for its stimulating effects. Daily requirement is 1-2 micrograms.

Pyridoxine or B_6 was established in 1936 as a separate vitamin B factor by Birch and Gyorgy. The compound was synthesized in 1939 by Harris and Folkers in the USA, and Kuhn and his group in Germany. Deficiency of this vitamin produces gastrointestinal disturbances and neuromuscular pain. Daily requirement is about 2 mg. Pyridoxine is employed to treat gastrointestinal disturbances, neuromuscular pains, nausea and vomiting of pregnancy, neuritis, pernicious vomiting, irradiation sickness, shingles, convulsions in vitamin B_6 deficient infants, some types of anemia and certain genetic disorders. There are other components of vitamin B.

Among them are choline, biotin, inositol, pantothenic acid, folic acid, and paraamino benzoic acid.

In 1912, Holst and Frolich postulated, as the result of guinea pig experiments, that the missing factor in scurvy was vitamin C. In this disease, there are hemorrhages of the skin and deeper tissues, changes in the skin, hair, and gums, poor wound healing, anemia, mental depression, and eventually death. Hess showed in his work between the years 1911-18 that this anti-scurvy factor was present in citrous fruit and tomatoes. The value of citrous fruit was known to Lind in the 18th century and the American Indians were aware of some curative factors in certain barks and leaves of trees. Szent-Gyorgi isolated ascorbic acid in 1927 without recognizing it was vitamin C. In 1932, King and Waugh proved that ascorbic acid was a vitamin C. Vitamin C is found in oranges, limes, grapefruit, lemons, cabbage, onions, turnips, ascerola, peppers, and other edibles. The daily requirement is usually stated to be 50-75 mg. Deficiency of vitamin C is manifested by prescorbic manifestations, scurvy, defective teeth formation.

Vitamin C is used to treat and prevent scurvy. It is administered also for fragility of blood capillaries, which rupture and bleed easily. It has been taken in large doses to prevent colds and respiratory infections. Wound healing and fractures knit slowly if there is a deficiency of ascorbic acid in the diet. Some types of anemia respond better if vitamin C is included in thearpy. This vitamin is an anti-oxidant and advocated as an agent to retard the aging process of the cell.

For a long time, the laity knew that cod liver oil cured rickets, but nobody knew why. Mellanby in 1918 and McCollum in 1924 demonstrated that a vitamin in cod liver oil was the essential curative substance, now known as vitamin D. In 1924, Steenbock, Hess, and Weinstock demonstrated that the curative effects of sunlight on rickets were due to the action of ultraviolet light on a fatty substance, ergosterol, in the skin. Later, pure vitamin D was isolated from irradiated ergosterol. Vitamin D is needed for metabolism of calcium and phosphorus, especially in growing children. When lacking, rickets ensues with bone malformation, waddling gait, weakness of muscles, and loss of appetite.

Other vitamins were discovered in time. Among the more important discoveries was that of vitamin K, by Henrik Dam in **1934**, which prevents hemorrhages. Lack of vitamin K prolongs clotting time. Another important vitamin is vitamin E which was discovered by Evans and Bishop in 1922. This vitamin is necessary for reproduction. Lack of it in the system results in sterility. Vitamin E is an antioxidant and as such is most important in delaying the aging process in cells. It is also used in large doses to treat angina and other heart disorders.

In 1912, Ernest von Behring (1854-1917) introduced a new vaccine for imunizing children against diphtheria, the so-called diphtheria toxin-antitoxin method. The prevalent method was to use diphtheria toxin alone, and, due to the potency of the toxin, there were many side effects. The new method eliminated most of these undesirable reactions. In 1892, along with Kisato, von Behring had prepared tetanus antitoxin, another great advance in medicine.

About this time Kronig and Gauss introduced the pain-relieving "twilight sleep" for women in labor. It was a combination of morphine and scopolamine, and it enjoyed an immense popularity for many years.

Few medical innovations were introduced in World War I (1914-1918). Antibiotics were unknown and, to combat sepsis in battle wounds, a preparation known as Carrell-Dakin solution was used. This solution liberated chlorine when introduced into wounds. Devitalized tissue was amputated before wounds were sewed up, thereby reducing sepsis also. Gas gangrene, a fatal disease if untreated, occurred frequently and was treated by an antitoxin developed by Bull. In this disorder, the infecting microbe often produce enormous quantities of gas in contaminated wounds. The sepsis destroyed tissues and gangrene followed.

Typhoid, paratyphoid, and cholera vaccines were given to troops to prevent these respective diseases. Delousing procedures were used to stop the spread of typhus by the ubiquitous infesting louse. Tetanus antitoxin was given to all wounded troops to cut down the mortality from tetanus infection in dirty battle wounds. This was the first war in which battle casualties were higher than disease morbidity.

New hormone discoveries came along. In 1915, Kendall isolated and crystallized the thyroid hormone, thyroxine. This was later synthesized in 1927. Long and Evans in 1921 showed that there was a growth hormone in the anterior or forward part of the pituitary gland. When there is an overproduction of this hormone, people develop overgrowth of bones, connective tissue and body organs. If this malfunction occurs in children, giants are produced. Thyroid, either whole gland or thyroxine, has been used to treat a patient whose gland is underfunctioning. Such a condition is known as hypothyroidism. Examples are goitre, where the oversize gland protrudes from the neck, myxedema in adults which is accompanied by thickening of the skin and mental sluggishness, or cretinism in children with physical and mental retardation. There is another hormone manufactured by the thyroid gland, namely triiodothyronine. Overdoses of thyroid hormones give rise to weight loss, goitre, fast heart beat, nervousness, tremors, and visual disturbances. The condition is known as hyperthyroidism. The activity of the thyroid gland is controlled by the thyrotropic hormone (thyroid stimulating hormone) elaborated by the pituitary gland. Recently a new hormone, calcitonin was isolated. It prevents excessive calcium levels and is antagonistic to parathormone which raises blood calcium levels.

The thyroid hormones are necessary for the normal functioning of the sex glands, carbohydrate metabolism, calcium levels in the blood, and general body metabolism. In hyperthyroidism, blood cholesterol levels are low and in hypothyroidism high. As a result, thyroid has been used to lower blood cholesterol. The most popular preparation utilized at present is sodium dextrothyroxine. Thyroid preparations can be given orally or by injection.

In 1917, Wagner von Jauregg, having been impressed by the disappearance of mental symptoms in psychotic patients suffering from typhoid fever, determined to try fever therapy in such cases. He finally accomplished his objective by injecting malaria-infected blood into patients suffering from syphilis of the brain, known as paresis. The experiment proved to be successful, and this method of treating neurosyphilis was quickly adopted around the world. Today, of course, penicillin is effective in the treatment of syphilis and fever therapy is now obsolete.

Another great psychiatrist was becoming quite famous in Vienna at this time. He was Sigmund Freud, the father of psychoanalysis.

During the years of 1918-1919, there was a world-wide epidemic of influenza, known as Spanish influenza. It was one of the worst epidemics ever recorded. Millions of people perished, civilians and military alike. Yet, the cause, method and spread, and effective treatment were mysteries and it was only much later, in 1933, that Smith, Andrews, and Laidlaw were able to demonstrate that a virus was the etological factor. In 1940, Magill and Francis discovered a second virus, which they called virus B, to distinguish it from virus A previously detected. Fearing a second epidemic, with all the tragedy attending that of World War I, a flu-virus vaccine was developed and administered to all American military personnel during World War II. Results were spectacularly successful. Since then, the vaccine has been improved periodically and now contains virus material from the "Hong Kong" flu variant which spread over the world in 1968-69.

In 1921, a great discovery was made by Banting and Best. They isolated the hormone insulin from the pancreas, and a new impetus for living was now available for moderate to severe sufferers of diabetes. With insulin, physicians could handle more successfully severe diabetes and also the dreaded diabetic coma with its high mortality. At first, it was felt that diabetes was due to faulty production of insulin by the body. In time, this was shown not to be the answer, because many other factors were involved in the etiology of diabetes, a disease in which the chief manifestation is a derangement of carbohydrate metabolism. Blood sugar (glucose) levels are high, and sugar may or may not always appear in the urine.

Common symptoms of diabetes are increased appetite, weight loss, thirst, hunger and increased urination. Special blood tests are available for making the diagnosis. The modalities for treating the diabetic patients are diet, insulin, exercise, and the orally-taken antidiabetic drugs. The latter are of two types, sulfonylureas and diguanides, and their method of action is not clearly understood. Jambon and Loubatieres discovered the antidiabetic sulfa drugs in 1942.

Insulin is the sheet anchor in diabetic therapy because of its ability to lower blood sugar levels and to increase the general metabolism of glucose. Insulin was formerly utilized to produce shock in certain mental patients. In very small doses, it may be used to stimulate the appetite and act as a general tonic. At one time it was used in this conjunction to heal duodenal and gastric ulcers.

Overdoses of insulin will produce low blood sugar levels and may result in "insulin shock" with symptoms of weakness, sweating, anxiety, flushing, pallor, and even convulsions, coma, and death. Orange juice, if given early, will counteract the low blood sugar and bring it back to safe levels. Insulin is a protein, and if given by mouth, will be destroyed by the digestive juices and therefore can only be given effectively by injection.

The female ovarian hormone, estrin, was detected by Allen and Doisy in 1923. Doisy and his co-workers crystallized out the hormone in 1930. Since that time, many estrogenic and progesterone derivatives have been elaborated by the pharmaceutical houses. Some are synthetic, others natural. Recent drugs produced are the birth control preparations, which are mostly synthetic and contain progesterone-like activity which inhibits ovulation.

The ovarian hormones are used for many purposes such as relieving the symptoms of the menopause (change-of-life), to prevent lactation (dry up a mother's milk), to relieve prostatic cancer in the male and breast cancer in the female, to ameliorate vaginitis in young girls and in the post-menopausal woman, and to ease the symptoms of senile vaginitis and itching of the external genitalia in older women. These hormones have also been utilized in men with coronary artery disease to prevent recurring heart attacks.

Side effects reported from the long continued use of the hormones are atrophy of the ovaries and disturbed calcium metabolism. Large doses may cause headaches, vomiting, and dizziness. Birth control pills frequently cause uncomfortable feelings, blotchy pigmentation of the skin, and occassionally abnormal blood clotting. These hormones may be given orally or by injection.

Koch and McGee isolated the male hormones from bull testes in 1927. They were finally identified as testosterone and androsterone in 1935 by Butenandt. Since that time, many derivatives have been synthesized as in the case of the female hormones.

Testosterone is used for hypogonadism (underfunctioning of the male sex glands), undescended testicles in young boys, the male climacteric (so called male change-of-life which is not similar to menopause in woman), menopause in women, female breast cancer, excessive bleeding from the uterus, and to dry up nursing breasts. It is also employed as an anabolic agent, as are chemical derivatives of this hormone, for increasing the buildup of body tissue and strength. Side effects are elevated blood calcium, flushing of the face, excessive hair growth on the body (hirsutism), deepening of the voice and acne in the female. The hormone is given by injection or orally.

In 1924, Calmette and Guerin prepared an anti-tuberculosis vaccine from live, non-virulent, tuberculosis germs of cattle. This bovine vaccine was used initially in France, and later in other parts of Europe, to immunize children against tuberculosis. The procedure was frowned upon in America for many years and then later received some trials. It has been recommended by some authorities for immunizing children in tuberculosis prone families. While effective vaccines have been developed for many diseases, this is not true for tuberculosis.

At the turn of the century, tuberculosis was the most frequent cause of death in the temperate zones and second only to malaria in the tropics. In the USA, tuberculosis was frequently transmitted from infected cows to man. Destruction of such herds eliminated this source of disease. Improvement of hygiene and sanitation has contributed to the decline of this dread disorder.

The most important treatment available in the early part of this century was lung surgery and pneumothorax, the introduction of air into the chest to rest the lung. They were widely employed in the 1930's. Following the introduction of the antibiotic streptomycin in 1945, such procedures fell into disrepute. Later, the introduction of isoniazide in 1952 revolutionized the treatment not only of pulmonary (lung) tuberculosis, but all form of the disease such as kidney, bone and joint. Later, PAS (paraminosalicylate) was added as an additional drug for treatment. Isoniazide has been considered the best medication. These drugs may be used singly or in combination. The most recent effective drugs are capreomycin, ethambutol, and rifamycin. They may be used singly or in combination.

In 1927, Ascheim and Zondek discovered the gonadotropic hormone (sex gland stimulating hormone) of the pituitary which controls the reproductive organs. This discovery led to the first good pregnancy test, the Ascheim Zondek Test.

In 1929, Corner and Allen demonstrated progesterone, the corpus luteum hormone of the ovary. This hormone enables the uterus to hold a pregnancy until term. If the hormone is not adequately produced miscarriage will ensue. Today, most progesterone hormones are prepared synthetically. Medical use is in the treatment of painful menstruation, excessive menstrual bleeding, threatened miscarriage, and birth control. Side effects are rare.

In 1934, Kendall isolated the adrenal hormone known as desoxycorticosterone, which made it possible now to treat Addison's disease, a deficiency in production of adrenal hormones. The disease is provoked by complete or partial destruction of the gland, caused by infection, cancer, or other conditions. Symptoms are weakness, low blood pressure, pigmentation of the skin, loss of weight, and decreased appetite.

In 1936, Mason, Myers, and Kendall discovered cortisone, another adrenal hormone. Hench found that this preparation was of value in Addison's disease, rheumatic fever, and rheumatoid arthritis. Soon there followed the uncovering of more adrenal hormones.

Remarkably, all secretions of the adrenal cortex, or outer portion of the gland, are chemically derived from cholesterol and therefore are called steroids. They are of three types—glucocorticoids which affect carbohydrate and protein metabolism, mineralocorticoids which affect water and mineral (electrolyte) metabolism, and the androgens which affect male sex characteristics.

Most fascinating are the glucocorticoids. They convert protein to carbohydrate which is deposited in the liver. They induce a loss of protein from many tissues and interfere with fat metabolism, resulting in patients developing fatty deposits in unusual areas such as the back (giving rise to a humpback appearance), the abdomen, and the face (creating a "moon face" look). Glucocorticoids cause swelling in tissues by retaining sodium and excreting potassium, thereby altering a delicate water balance. These hormones reduce inflammation in tissues and shrink swollen glands (medically called nodes), as well as normal ones. The mineralocorticoids act like the glucocorticoids with relation to minerals, protein and fat metabolism. The androgens may be used in males or females if the need arises.

The corticosteroids have been found useful in allergy, rheumatoid arthritis, and asthma. Their most common employment is in reducing inflammatory reactions in various disorders. They are life saving in Addison's disease and may be used in overwhelming infections along with antibiotics. The corticosteroids are frequently utilized in treating tuberculosis, especially in Europe, to stop the destructive effects of the tuberculosis germ. They have been used, also, to prevent rejection of transplanted organs.

Side and toxic effects of the steroids are many. There is swelling and rounding of the face known as "moon face," along with an increase in weight, and abnormal deposits of fat. Appetite is more marked. Scalp hair becomes thinner while body hair is more noticeable. Acne and pigmentation may appear. Blood pressure increases and the heart rate is accelerated. Due to the anti-inflammatory effect there is low resistance to infection. Wounds and fractures heal slowly. Blood sugar rises. Stomach and duodenal ulcers may rupture. Mental symptoms may appear. Among the steroid drugs available are a number of natural and synthetic hormones. They are cortisone, hydrocortisone, prednisone, prednisolone, aldosterone, desoxycorticosterone, dexamethasone, fluorinated and other derivatives.

In 1942, ACTH (adreno-corticotropic hormone) was isolated by Li, Evans, and Simpson, along with Sayers, White and Long. The discovery marked another important advance in medicine. This pituitary hormone stimulates the adrenal gland to pour out its hormones. ACTH is used in a similar manner to the adrenal hormones in medicine. It has the same side effects. Li, who isolated ACTH, also found STH (somatropic hormone) the growth hormone of the pituitary which can be used to treat stunted growth.

One of the most dramatic discoveries in all of medicine occurred in this century, and that is the story of the antibiotics. We can, in fact, call this the "Century of the Antibiotics." At the beginning of the twentieth century, specific medications such as quinine and ipecac were available only against the protozoan diseases of malaria and amebic dysentery. In 1910, Ehrlich synthesized the first anti-infectious drug, salvarsan.

In the evolutionary scheme of things, living microscopic organisms learned to exist by killing off their adversaries by physical violence or chemical means. At this time, we are interested mainly in their chemical warfare. The antagonism of living microbes for one another was first noticed by Pasteur in 1877. Vuillemin in 1889 devised the term "antibiosis" to indicate this chemical phenomenon. In 1898, Rudolph Emmerich, a German bacteriologist, found that an extract from a microbe called pyocyaneus, now known as pseudomonas aeruginosa, would kill the organisms which caused diphtheria, typhoid fever, and anthrax. This very promising phenomenon failed to have practical value, for the substance was too toxic for human therapy. The ancient Chinese and the American Indians used mold extracts for superficial infections and the medical literature over the centuries records the beneficial effects of soil or plants applied to infections, presumably due to presence of germ killing chemicals elaborated by soil bacteria and molds. The discovery of antibiotics was bound to happen sooner or later. It was a fact looking for a discoverer. In 1917, German investigators noted that certain compounds, used as dyes in Germany and known as sulfonamides, could kill microbes. But nothing came out of this finding until Gerhard Domagk in 1935 observed that the red dye prontosil protected mice against fatal streptococcal induced infection. The actual substance in the prontosil molecule was sulfanilamide. The drug was found to be effective against erysipelas, septic sore throat (streptococcus throat), puerperal sepsis of pregnancy, and meningitis.

Rapidly, the chemists went to work to find other sulfa drugs that might be more potent. In 1938, Whitby in England synthesized sulfapyridine which was effective against pneumonia and staphylococcus infections. However, in 1939, the American drug sulfathiazole, introduced by Perrin Long, replaced sulfapyridine due to its greater effectiveness against pneumonia. Then came sulfadiazine, introduced by Richard Roblin in 1940, one of the best sulfa drugs ever synthesized. It was quite effective against meningitis and other disorders. Derivatives of sulfathiazole, such as succinyl sulfathiazole, were used to combat intestinal infection because they remained in the gut and were largely unabsorbed.

The sulfa drugs were found to be of local antiseptic value and were put into war wounds before they were sewed up during the World War II period. They were also placed into the abdomen in cases of peritonitis as well as being given orally. Sulfa drugs were given before tooth extraction in cases of valvular diseases of the heart, so that organisms getting into the blood stream would not be able to lodge on these diseased valves and give rise to bacterial endocarditis.

Over the following decades, new sulfa drugs were introduced, some of them stood the test of time, others like the older sulfa drugs fell into disuse. In general the sulfa drugs are considered anti-infective and are especially valuable in combating organisms such as pneumococci, streptococci, staphylococci, meningococci, gonococci, clostridium tetani and welchii, and others. These microbes produce such disorders as pneumonia; throat and skin infections; sinus infections and bronchitis; meningitis, gonorrhea, tetanus, gas gangrene, peritonitis, arthritis, and urinary and kidney infections.

The sulfa drugs are usually given by mouth. The soluble ones are quickly absorbed, others are relatively insoluble and are valuable for local antiseptic action in the bowel. The method of action of these compounds is not fully understood. It is believed that the microbes absorb them into their metabolism in place of certain normal substances thereby weakening or killing themselves.

Toxic or side reactions resulting from sulfa ingestion are nausea, vomiting, light headedness, dizziness, fatigue, exhaustion, depression, skin rashes, fever, jaundice and adverse reactions of the blood cells.

The treatment of diseases with sulfa drugs is known as chemotherapy. Among the commonly used sulfa drugs today are sulfadimethoxine (Madribon®), a long acting anti-infective preparation; sulfisomidine (Elkosin®), an anti-infective drug; succinylsulfathiazole (Sulfasuxidine®), poorly absorbed and used in intestinal infections and intestinal operations; sulfamethizole (Thiosulfil®), a urinary antiseptic; sulfacetamide (Sulamyd®), an antiseptic; sulfameter (Sulla®), a general anti-infective preparation; sulfamethoxazole (Gantanol®), a urinary antiseptic and general anti-infectious agent; sulfisoxazole (Gantrisin®), a urinary antiseptic. The names enclosed in parentheses are proprietary names for the product put out by specific pharmaceutical houses.

Next to appear on the scene were the antibiotics, so called because they were elaborated by micro-organism instead of chemists. Actually, chemotherapy is antibiotic too, for it destroys living organisms and the distinction is purely academic. The fascinating saga of antibiotics began one day in 1928. Fleming, a British bacteriologist, was growing germ cultures in his laboratory. One of these became contaminated by a mold, just like cut fruit exposed to the air. The strange thing Fleming noted, was that the germs were killed by this contaminant, a mold called penicillium. This occurrence and serendipitous observation provided physicians eventually with one of the greatest medical discoveries of all time.

However, it took ten years before intensive research work followed this observation. W. H. Florey and Ernest Chain of Britain came to the U.S.A. in 1941 for help in producing penicillin from the penicillium mold. A massive effort was undertaken with the help of the United States Government, resulting in large quantities of penicillin being produced for the armed forces in World War II.

By the end of the war there was enough available for military and civilian needs.

Penicillin and the sulfa drugs helped to overcome many infectious diseases. Bacterial pneumonia had had a death rate of about 30 percent. Sulfa drugs cut the mortality rate to 10 percent and penicillin to less than 5 percent. All infectious diseases did not respond, unfortunately, to these two agents. However, new antibiotics were on the horizon, waiting to be discovered.

Different types of penicillin have been marketed over the years and, even today, new preparations are being brought out. Penicillin is made in a number of types such as F,G,K,O,V.X, but G is the most common and is said to be the most potent. Penicillin can be given either by mouth or injection. It is effective against streptococci, pneumococci, staphylococci, gonococci, meningococci, clostridium tetani and welchii, the treponema of syphilis, some fungi and other organisms. The diseases caused by these organisms were enumerated with the sulfa drugs.

Among the types of penicillin available are crystalline potassium penicillin G; procaine penicillin G; penicillin V; synthetic penicillins for staphylococcus resistance infections; ampicillin and other broad spectrum penicillins.

Penicillin is bactericidal (kills bacteria), and also bacteriostatic (impedes the growth of bacteria). Its method of activity is presumed to be due to blocking the synthesis of the bacterial wall. Toxic and side effects are uncommon. However, allergic reactions may occur and these may be mild, severe, or even lethal. Sometimes penicillin is blamed for reactions which are due to the vehicle in which it is given and not the drug itself.

The American, Selman Waksman, in 1939 directed his attention to soil bacteria, looking for a drug to kill the tuberculosis germ. In view of the fact that the microbe is rapidly killed when buried, Waksman felt he might find the answer in the ground. After 5 years and 10,000 species of soil bacteria he came up with streptomycin in 1944, the first anti-tuberculosis drug. It was derived from a bacterial group known as the streptomyces, which later gave rise to other antibiotics including the "broad spectrum" tetracyclines which attack a wide range of bacteria. Waksman, incidentally, coined the term "antibiotic."

Bacteria are usually classified as gram positive or gram negative, depending upon their staining abilities. Penicillin is mostly active against gram positive organisms such as streptococci, staphylococci, pneumococci, clostridia, and others, but also is effective against a few gram negative organisms as the gonococcus and meningococcus. Streptomycin, on the contrary, is active against gram negative microbes such as the colon bacillus, which lives in the bowel, and germs causing tularemia and brucellosis. Until recent times, penicillin and streptomycin were combined in one injection to get a broad spectrum of response against infection, especially where the nature of the organism was unknown.

Streptomycin is either lethal or inhibitory to susceptible bacteria by disrupting their metabolism. Unfortunately the drug has a serious fault which has been slowly sending it into limbo. It frequently produces deafness. Toxic symptoms and side reactions noted are vertigo, dizziness, skin rashes, fever, and joint discomfort.

Other drugs have been developed from the streptomyces family. One of these, dihydrostreptomycin, is more toxic than the parent drug and is less frequently. Like the original medication, it can only be given by injection. Kanamycin (Kantrex®) reacts against gram positive and negative organisms. It is effective against the staphylococcus and is given mainly by injection. It must be used cautiously because it may cause deafness and kidney damage. Neomycin is poorly absorbed from the bowel. It is prescribed orally for diarrheas of infectious origin. Because of the fact that it may cause deafness and kidney damage it is seldom used by injection, and then only if no other antibiotic is effective. However, the drug is used topically for local infections of the skin. There is one other drug in this class, paromomycin, and it has been used for bowel infections.

Chloramphenicol (Chloromycetin®) was isolated in 1947 by Burkholder from a strain of streptomyces living in the soil of Venezuela, and studied by John Ehrlich in 1948. It is one of the most versatile of all antibiotics and effective against many gram positive and gram negative bacteria. It is very valuable especially in the treatment of typhoid and typhus fever, Rocky Mountain spotted fever, the Japanese river fever known as tsutsugamushi disease or scrub typhus.

The last three diseases are caused by a class of germs known as Rickettsia. They were named after their discoverer, the American Howard Ricketts, who died himself from Mexican typhus in 1910 at the age of 39 while studying this disorder. The Rickettsial organisms

Drugs, Demons, Doctors, and Disease

exist in the gut of lice, fleas, ticks, and mites. Rocky Mountain fever is produced by the bite of ticks, Japanese River Fever by the bite of mites, and Typhus fever by the bite of human lice or rat-transmitted fleas.

Typhus fever is characterized by a high fever, severe headache, and a skin rash. Typhus epidemics, especially in eastern Europe, have killed millions of people. In wartime, typhus has frequently been the deciding factor. With the discovery and use of chloramphenicol, the typhus scourge could be licked for the first time in human history.

Chloramphenicol, more popularly known as Chloromycetin®, was the first potent drug against brucellosis, a disease transmitted to man by the goat, pig, or cow. The organism producing the disease is called brucella. The most characteristic symptom of the disease is the fever which alternates with periods of normal temperature. This febrile undulation has been responsible for the condition often being called undulant fever. Other anti-brucellosis drugs are the tetracyclines, streptomycin, and the sulfas.

Chloromycetin® is of value in the treatment of such venereal diseases as chancroid, which also responds to the sulfas and tetracyclines; granuloma inguinale, which responds to the tetracyclines; and gonorrhea which responds to penicillin, tetracyclines, and sulfa. The dysenteries caused by the shigella and salmonella organisms are successfully treated by chloromycetin. Tularemia, transmitted by infected rodents, is treated by this drug as well as with tetracyclines.

Toxic and side effects of chloromycetin are nausea, vomiting, gastrointestinal discomfort, diarrhea, drug rashes, and rarely blood cell disorders. In one out of 150,000 people treated with this drug a fatal blood disorder may occur. This is due to depression of cells in the bone marrow. As a result of this rare reaction, it has been suggested that chloromycetin be used only when no other antibiotic is effective.

The tetracyclines are a very valuable addition to the armamentarium of physicians for fighting infection. The earliest ones to be discovered and used were chlortetracycline (Aureomycin®) in 1948 and oxytetracycline (Terramycin®) in 1950, both derived from different streptomyces soil bacteria. From a mutation of the Aureomycin producing streptomyces in 1959 came another excellent drug, demethylchlortetracycline (Declomycin®).

These drugs are known as broad spectrum antibiotics because they cover a wide range of activity against bacteria and some viruses. The tetracyclines are used singly or questionably sometimes in combination with penicillin. The efficacy of these drugs varies with the particular preparation. In general, they are utilized with good results in treating Rickettsial diseases such as typhus fever, Q fever, and Rocky Mountain Spotted fever; infections of the respiratory and urinary tracts; venereal diseases; large viruses which cause psittacosis (a bird-transmitted disease) and trachoma (an eye disease); amebic infestations. Tetracyclines probably exert their action by interfering with bacterial metabolism.

These drugs are usually administered by mouth. The toxicity and side effects are mainly associated with the stomach and bowel. There may be nausea, heartburn, vomiting, and diarrhea. Allergic reactions are seen occasionally. Declomycin® is associated with light sensitivity, and, in some patients, exposure to sunlight while taking the medication may cause skin rashes.

The preparations available are chlortetracycline (Aureomycin®), demethylchlortetracycline (Declomycin®), doxycycline (Vibramycin®), methacycline (Rondomycin®), oxytetracycline (Terramycin®), tetracycline (Achromycin®, Steclin®, Pancycin®), tetracycline phosphate complex (Tetrex®, Sumycin®, Tetracyn®, Panmycin Phosphate®).

A new type of antibiotic, erythromycin, was isolated in 1952 from a type of streptomyces by McGuire and his coworkers. It is effective against streptococci, staphylococci, and pneumococci. It frequently destroys staphylococci that are resistant to penicillin. Preparations available are Erythrocin®, E-Mycin®, Bristamycin® and Ilosone®. Toxic and side effects are chiefly gastrointestinal, allergies are rare.

Another group of antibiotics are derived from the bacillus polymyxa also called aerosporus. They are called polymyxins, and designated as A, B, C, D, and E. The B and E are the least toxic and so are used medically. Polymyxin E is marketed as colistin (Coly-Mycin®) and was discovered by the Japanese in 1950. These drugs are highly effective against gram negative organisms. Their method of action is believed to be due to altering the permeability of the bacterial cell walls. Polymyxins are only used by injection when other antibiotics are not effective, for they can damage nerves and kidneys. They are not absorbed from the gut. The polymyxins are useful for topical application to local infections often being combined with bacitracin (derived from the subtilis bacillus), which exerts an activity against gram positive microbes.

Gentamycin (Garamycin®), produced by the micromonospora organism, has a wide bacterial spectrum. It is toxic and seldom used by injection. It is mostly employed for topical use. The same is true for tyrothrycin, derived from the soil bacillus brevis.

Other antibiotics which are used on occasion are Lincomycin®, Oleandomycin®, Ristocetin®, Vancomycin®, Viomycin®, Nitrofurantoin®.

Among the important advances made in antibiotic development were those directed against fungus infections. Nystatin (Mycostatin®), isolated from streptomyces noursei from the soil of Virginia in 1951 by Hazen and Brown, is active against the fungus candida, also known as monilia, which causes infections of the mucus membranes, skin, vagina, and gastrointestinal tract. Thrush is seen in infants, and is a mouth infection caused by candida. Vaginal candida involvement is especially noted during pregnanacy, while intestinal infection is seen in debilitated patients. Nystatin is applied locally in oral or vaginal infection and is given by mouth for gut involvement. It is not absorbed from the intestinal tract.

Another valuable antifungal antibiotic is amphotericin B (Fungizone®). It is derived from a soil organism known as streptomyces nodosus found in the Orinoco River region of Venezuela. There is an A and B variety, but the latter is the most valuable in fighting certain types of fungal infection. Like nystatin, it is effective against candida infections and useful in combating San Joaquin Valley disease of California (known also by its medical name of coccidioidomycosis) a lung infection by the fungus coccidoides. Amphotericin B is used against both North and South American blastomycoses in which the blastomyces fungus invades the skin, mucus membranes and internal organs. The drug can also be used against histoplasmosis, an internal fungal infection, as well as protozoal infections. It can only be given intravenously. The drug has side effects which may be toxic and dangerous. Kidney damage is a common complication. Like nystatin, amphotericin B probably acts by damaging the cell walls of fungi, protozoa, and animals.

The discovery of griseofulvin added another antifungal agent to our defensive armamentarium. Griseofulvin was isolated from a mold known as penicillium griseofulvum by Oxford in 1939. It was ineffective against bacteria and so was discarded. In 1946, Brian found a substance in another penicillium organism which was antifungal. In analyzing this reaction they found the active component was griseofulvin. It should be mentioned at this point that regular penicillin does not have any griseofulvin action. For 10 years, griseofulvin was used to treat fungus diseases of cattle. Finally, in 1958, Gentles discovered that the drug could cure fungus infections of the feet in humans.

Griseofulvin is active against fungal organisms which produce infections of the feet, commonly referred to as 'Athletes Foot." It is not active against candida infections or the white-spotted fungal disease of the skin known medically as tinea versicolor. It is also ineffective against internal fungal infections. Griseofulvin's main action is directed against superficial fungal infections of the skin and nails. The drug is fungistatic (inhibits fungal growth) but does not kill the organisms. Side effects noted are gastrointestinal discomfort and diarrhea. The drug is given orally. Preparations available are Grisactin®, Fulvicin®, and Grifulvin®.

There is one type of fungus infection that responds to penicillin and is called actinomycosis. In this disease there is involvement of the face, neck, chest, and abdomen. During the early years of this century, actinomycosis was the commonest internal fungal disease. Other antibiotics may be of supplemental help in treating the disorders. The sulfa drugs are of value in treating nocardiosis, a fungal disease of the respiratory tract.

For most disease-producing organisms, there is usually one drug or occasionally a number of drugs that may be used to achieve maximum effectiveness with a reasonable degree of safety. If the patient does not respond to treatment as expected, or cannot tolerate the initial medication, alternative preparations may be used. Con sequently there are first choice drugs and alternates in most cases.

If time is of the essence, the physician will prescribe a drug he feels is the best possible choice. If the situation demands further investigation, an attempt will be made to identify the infecting organism. Then, sensitivity tests will be performed with various antibiotics and chemotherapeutic agents to find the drug or drugs best suited to fight the infection.

However, because this is a world in which things are often not what they seem, an organism other than the one responsible for the disorder may be isolated and treatment consequently directed towards this microbe does not help the prime situation. An additional situation may arise in which an insufficient dosage of the correct drug may prove ineffective in overcoming the infecting organism. Poor host resistance to the infection may further handicap correct treatment. Sometimes an antimicrobial agent, which on testing may appear to be relatively inactive, will be effective when administered. If one drug, on the basis of tests, does not secure the desired results when prescribed, another will have to be tried. In tuberculosis and certain enterococcal infections of the heart, more than one antibiotic may be used from the beginning of therapy.

At this point, we shall look at the strange bits of life known as viruses. The great discoveries of the 1940s and 1950s gave physicians a well-stocked arsenal of antibacterial weapons. But the viruses for the most part resisted these drugs. Vaccines have markedly reduced the incidence of viral diseases such as polio, smallpox, influenza, measles, and rubella. The unvaccinated individual, however, is helpless and can depend upon no drugs but only his own resistance in fighting off these viral infections. This is also true of other viral diseases of the respiratory tract, gut, the brain in encephalitis and the liver in hepatitis.

One reason for the slow progress in challenging the viruses is that they were difficult to study in the laboratories until recently. Again, their biological structure is very simple which makes them harder to attack lethally. The simplest bacteria need hundreds of chemical reactions to exist and any drug which can alter or block these actions can have a static or killing effect. The viral metabolic processes require very few reactions and these have not been seriously altered by drugs as yet.

The largest viruses are actually at the level of the smallest bacteria and hence more complex than the very small or simple viruses. They may respond to the tetracyclines or erythromycin. Such is the mycoplasma pneumoniae which causes primary or atypical pneumonia. The agent of psittacosis, a bird and fowl transmitted disease, repsonds to tetracycline and chloromycetin; lymphogranuloma venereum, a venereal disease, yields to tetracyclines and chloromycetin; herpes simplex, the common "cold sore" virus, when it infects the eye may respond to an iodine compound known as idoxuridine.

At present there are no available drugs to kill the smaller viruses. The respiratory viruses such as the rhino, myxo, influenza (A and B, Asian, parainfluenza) adeno, syncytial, corona, reo, RS, and others are far more common invaders of the nose, throat, and chest than the bacteria. These organisms cause many common illnesses such as the common cold, sinusitis, tonsillitis, pharyngitis including croup, tracheo-bronchitis, and pneumonia (medically known as pneumonitis). Frequently, as the result of the host's resistance being down sharply as the result of the viral onslaught, a secondary invasion may follow with disease-producing bacteria. These may have been dormant in the body or they may be new ones which are introduced at this time. In epidemics of the flu, many times death is due to secondary invading microorganisms. In these patients, antibiotics become lifesaving agents.

Our best defense today against viruses is immunization. The earliest successful vaccination was against smallpox in the eighteenth century by Jenner. Pasteur in 1885 introduced the rabies anti-vaccine. In the 20th century vaccines have been developed against yellow fever by Max Theiler in 1937; polio by Jonas Salk in 1959 and Albert Sabin in 1961; influenza in World War II; measles by John Enders in 1961; mumps by Jeryl Hilleman in 1964; rubella (German measles) in 1969.

Viruses have been implicated in cancer. When one considers that to date more than 500 distinct types of viruses have been identified within the human body, with 40 to 60 causing the so called common cold, and because of their ability to invade the cell nucleus and merge with it, one can understand their ability to misdirect the normal cellular control mechanism. In 1898, Beijerinck demonstrated the tobacco mosaic virus that destroyed the tobacco plant. In 1911, Peyton Rous showed that a virus caused a cancer in chickens.

There is now known to be cancer viruses. Leukemia has been identified with viruses. The so called EB (Epstein-Barr) virus which causes infectious mononucleosis (the "Kissing Disease" of young people) was identified in 1968 with Burkitt's lymphoma, a form of cancer in Africans. We are all exposed to this virus. In most people the infection is harmless, in others the "Kissing Disease" develops, and in a few susceptible individuals cancer makes its appearance. Cancer of the womb is believed to be closely related to the herpes virus, which is found in the smega (discharge under the foreskin) of uncircumcised males. It has been claimed by some authorities that women who engage in promiscuous sexual intercourse are more susceptible to cancer of the womb, because they have more contact with the herpes virus.

A virus vaccine has been prepared which will prevent experimental leukemia in mice. A vaccine prepared against the EB virus may prevent the Kissing Disease and also malignancies attributed to it. Cytoxan®, an anticancer drug, showed striking success against Burkitt's lymphomas in 1969. A vaccine against adenoviruses has proven to be quite effective when used by the armed forces. A vaccine against the syncytial viruses is about ready. This organism has been implicated in causing half the virus deaths from pneumonia in children each year.

A major goal of researchers, in addition to bringing out new virus vaccines, is to find drugs to curb these microbes. Amantadine, an A_2 virus preventer for exposed individuals, was brought out by duPont in 1968. Its full effectiveness is still to be determined. Interestingly, a patient with Parkinson's disease was given this drug when she had the flu. The improvement in her Parkinson's symptoms was so striking, that investigators gave the drug to other patients with this disease with equally satisfactory results. In 1962, Herbert Kaufman reported the successful use of idoxuridine in treating herpes simplex virus infections of the eye. In 1964, British researchers developed a drug called thiosemicarbazone which prevents smallpox in exposed individuals.

Perhaps the most promising approach to curbing virus infection is the discovery of interferon by Drs. Jean Lindenmann and Alick Isaacs in England in 1957. The DNA (deoxyribonucleic acid, a nucleic acid of cell nucleii) or RNA (ribonucleic acid, a cellular nucleic acid) of attacking viruses stimulates the infected cell to produce this protein, called interferon, which is carried by the blood stream to other cells and protects them against the viruses. Some investigators believe that interferon is more important than the antiviral antibodies in fighting viruses, although the antibodies are the major factor in preventing recurrences.

Because of the large amounts of interferon needed to fight disease, the administration of the natural substance, which is in short supply, is impossible at the present time. Researchers are working avidly on a way to solve the deficiency. They have found that injecting natural or synthetic RNA in animals induces interferon production. It has also been learned that certain chemicals may also stimulate cells to make interferon. Some of these preparations produce toxic and serious side effects. However, future research looks promising for these investigative attempts.

When infecting organisms invade the body, complex processes come into play, some of which we are aware of and perhaps some waiting to be discovered. Fever and inflammation are frequently observed. White cells, known as polys (polymorphonuclear leukocytes), attack and digest bacteria. Other white cells known as lymphs (lymphocytes) play a role in chronic infections and in producing antibodies. There are wandering cells known as macrophages which also engulf bacteria. To aid in infection control a substance known as complement is present in the blood to soften up bacteria for antibody attacks. Antibiotics are helpful in interfering with bacterial metabolism and reproduction, thereby enabling the natural body-defensive-mechanism to overcome the infection more easily. If the defenses are low or in a state of collapse, the results of antibiotic therapy will be poor or entirely ineffective.

The struggle for existence is keen among all life forms. It is especially true among microbic organisms. The fittest and most adaptable survive. Bacteria, and viruses also, may adopt to coexistence, or the more powerful forms may decimate or eliminate the weaker. A few bacteria of a particular group, which are susceptible to a specific antibiotic, may survive the administered antibiotic and their progeny will also become resistant to it. Where bacteria are living together in an uneasy truce and their numbers are kept down by mutual antibiosis, the killing off of one group by an antibiotic allows the remaining organism to grow uninhibited and a new problem arises for the host.

To complicate things a bit further, bacteria assume various patterns in culture growth. Usually they adopt recognizable forms. It has been found that they may assume another display, after treatment with antibiotics or when present in the body for a while. This pattern is called by various names, the most popular being L-form or L-variant, the "L" being derived from the initial letter of the Lister Institute of London, England, where the initial discovery was made in 1935. These forms, however, may revert back to their classical configurations when conditions are reversed. Carl Godzeski found that blood or other body fluids, enzymes, and antibodies cause the normal microbic forms to change to the L-form, presumably so that the body will be better able to cope with the invaders. In this new phase, the organisms lose their rigid walls and become soft forms. It is believed that the body enzyme, lysozyme, digests off the bacterial wall making the germ more susceptible to attack by the phagocytes which can then more easily engulf them.

Some investigators on the other hand believe that the soft and hard forms are only different phases in the growth of bacteria. Be that as it may, researchers have found in some cases that the organisms are sensitive to one antibiotic in one phase of their existence and to another in the succeeding phase. Chronic infections may be maintained, therefore, by microbes moving from one existence to another to escape antibiotic and immune mechanism attacks.

When measured against human misery, suffering, disease, and death there is little doubt that the discovery of chemotherapy and antibiotic therapy constitutes the most spectacular medical finding of all time. It is so dramatic because it has saved millions of people from premature death, shortened or prevented hospital confinements, and reduced economic hardships by preventing long periods of disability and eventual death from chronic infectious disease. Millions of people are alive today who would have been dead if it were not for antibacterial therapy.

Of course there have been many other important drug advancements in this century and we shall get to them soon, discussing them in relation to their particular field of use. We shall close this chapter with a final addition to the antibacterial discussions.

Less spectacular, but playing an important role in fighting infection, is the utilization of disinfectants and antiseptics. Because of common usage, the term disinfectant has become synonymous with germicide and bactericide, and it means a chemical which will kill all microbes. Originally the word meant a chemical which would kill disease-producing organisms. An antiseptic is a substance which inhibits the growth of microorganisms.

Most chemicals used for their antiseptic or disinfectant qualities are standarized by government rules and regulations. Some of these substances have a wide application while others may be quite restrictive.

An old time preparation which may be considered a mild and not very efficient disinfectant is soap. When used with water, soap has a washing or detergent action. This characteristic results in the physical removing of dirt and germs from a surface. Soap and water have been used to clean the skin before surgery and also for cleansing dirty wounds. The soapy mixture lowers the surface tension of bacteria and thus retards growth.

Some synthetic detergents have disinfectant action and are used on the skin. In addition they are employed to sterilize surgical instruments and for washing walls, floors, furniture, and other objects in hosiptals. Like soap, they lower surface tension of bacteria. Commonly used detergents for these purposes are benzalkonium chloride (Zephiran®, Benzalkone®), benzethonium chloride (Phemerol®), and cetyl pyridium chloride (Ceepryn®).

One of the most famous disinfectants is phenol. We have alluded to it in discussing Lister's asepsis in the nineteenth century which earned this surgeon a niche in medical history. Phenol, also known as carbolic acid, and phenol-type preparations are excellent disinfectants. Phenol, itself, has been used to sterilize wounds, the appendix stump after surgery, vaccines, and instruments. It has also been used as a skin cauterizing agent, a local skin anesthetic, and in skin chemexfoliation (chemosurgery, skin peeling). Phenol and its derivatives have been utilized in sewage and environmental disinfection.

Other phenol products are Lysol® and Kresol® which are saponated cresol solutions. They are widely employed in the home and hospitals. A very famous skin disinfectant is hexachlorophene known as Phisohex®.

Chlorine and Iodine, the so-called halogen chemicals, are excellent bactericidal agents. Chlorine is widely used as a disinfectant, especially for drinking and swimming pool water. Iodine is mostly employed as a surface sterilizing agent, especially on the skin, or in skin wounds.

In the past, dyes were employed as antiseptics and disinfectants. They have been mostly discarded. Still surviving are gentian violet, scarlet red, and acriflavine.

Mercury and Silver compounds have been considered as being good antiseptics and disinfectants. Well known mercury preparations are merbromin (Mercurochrome®), thiomerosal (Merthiolate®), nitromersol (Metaphen®), yellow oxide of mercury, and ammoniated mercury. Commonly used silver compounds have been silver nitrate and silver protein (Argyrol®). A few of these mercury and silver preparations have been felt to be of questionable value by some authorities.

Oxidizing agents, such as hydrogen peroxide, destroy germs by liberating oxygen, which is detrimental to organisms which are anerobic (live best in an environment containing little or no oxygen). Other frequently prescribed oxidizing chemicals are potassium permanganate, which makes a purplish solution and stains the skin brown, and sodium perborate.

There is a miscellaneous group of antiseptics and disinfectants. Among these are boric acid (which is rapidly going out of use), formaldehyde (utilized in preserving tissue specimens and also as embalming fluid), acetone and ether, alcohol, and nitrofuraxone (Furacin®). New products are coming out continuously. Many authorities consider 70% alcohol as being the best skin disinfectant.

In looking forward to medications which will come into use during this decade, a most interesting substance is prostaglandin, so called because it was first found in the prostate gland. Later, it was discovered in all human and animal tissue.

Actually, there is more than one type of prostaglandin. So far, 14 have been isolated, and 13 occur in man with the highest concentration being in the seminal fluid. The story of their discovery goes back to 1930 when Kurzok and Lieb noted that fresh human semen had the power to either contract or relax strips of human uterus. Goldblatt and von Euler are credited with being the co-discoverers of prostaglandin around 1935. Bergstrom isolated the pure crystalline form in 1957. Most of the research with these ubiquitous agents has been done in the last 10 years. At present, intense activity is going on with these substances in investigative centers all over the world.

These exciting prostaglandins can perform many activities such as inducing labor, producing abortion, preventing conception, treating male sterility, preventing peptic ulcers and thromboses (blood clots), healing peptic ulcers, lowering high blood pressure, opening constricted bronchial tubes in asthma, relieving nasal congestion. Many more mysteries of the prostaglandins are still to be unraveled.

For producing abortion or inducing labor, the prostaglandins may be given by vaginal suppository, by direct introduction in the uterus, intravenously, or by mouth. The interval between medication and abortion is relatively short and without serious side effects. The pituitary hormone oxytocin plays a role in inducing labor. Karim, a leading researcher in this field, suggests that prostaglandins and oxytocin act together to start the process or possibly oxytocin may release prostaglandin or vice versa. In any event, prostaglandin is found in the amniotic fluid, which surrounds the unborn child, and also in the venous blood of the mother during labor.

Prostaglandins also aid in the formation of cyclic AMP (adenosine monophosphate) and either turns it on or off in the cells. Cyclic AMP is the second messenger-system in the cells, the first being the prostaglandins. It mediates most if not all hormone actions in cells. This substance in some way releases insulin, histamine, pituitary and thyroid hormones, and is involved in liver metabolism, gastric secretion, and blood platelet aggregation in the blood, and other functions waiting to be discovered. High levels of cyclic AMP in blood platelets prevent blood from clotting whereas low levels are conducive to clotting (thromboses) within the blood vessels. Exciting speculations are current as to what valuable treatment possibilities will arise in the future from the use of prostaglandins, cyclic AMP, and other intriguing agents now being discovered and researched.

Chapter Seven

PREVENTIVE DRUGS

THE IDEAL GOAL OF THE MEDICAL PROFESSION is to prevent disease rather than treat it. Complete fulfillment of this most worthy ambition is yet to be achieved. But we have made considerable progress along the craggy, tortuous, and vexing road to wipe out sickness.

A number of methods have been adopted to prevent disease. The most ancient is to avoid or quarantine a sick person and to disinfect or destroy all articles used by this individual. The more fruitful plans call for administration of medication, the stimulation of the body to provide an active immunity, or, in an immediate emergency, to confer a temporary passive immunity.

In trying to ward off illness, the best prescription is to start with good health, a possession not universally shared by everyone. When one thinks of maintaining a good health routine, one automatically considers a proper diet, containing adequate amounts of proteins, fats, carbohydrates, minerals, and vitamins. Authorities may differ as to what "proper" diet is best, each having his own pet ideas. In addition to diet a moderate amount of exercise is considered essential, with no universal agreement as to what "moderate" actually is. A philosophy of equanimity for a lifetime of good health is advisable. Even if all these suggestions are met, one does not necessarily qualify for immunity to disease.

Bacteria, playfully called "bugs" by physicians, are no respecters of health, financial position, or political power. They are democratic in pursuing their careers and do not care whom they infect. However, a person in good health, has a marked advantage in combating a disease over one having poor health.

A number of prophylactic medications are available for fighting off sicknesses. In the last chapter we mentioned two drugs, amantadine and thiosemicarbazone, which are used to prevent A_2 influenza and smallpox respectively. Drugs like Aralen®, Atabrine®, and Daraprin® have been administered to troops in the South Pacific and Southeast Asia to prevent malaria. Antibiotics may be given to persons exposed to virulent bacterial diseases to which they have not been immunized. This procedure would apply to conditions such as typhoid and typhus fever, cholera, bubonic plague, fungus infections, and large virus infections such as mycoplasma or atypical pneumonia, psittacosis, and lymphogranuloma.

Exposure to childhood diseases such as diphtheria and scarlet fever would call for prophylactic antibiotic therapy. The same would be true for individuals exposed to venereal disorders, septic sore throat (streptococcus infections), meningitis, tetanus, and similar serious disorders.

Less serious illnesses also call for preventive treatment. In the so-called goitre belts around the world and in the Great Lakes region of the USA, there is a deficiency of iodide in the drinking water and soil. Administration of iodides prevents the development of endemic goitre. Fluorides are put into water in regions where it is low to deter dental caries. Antihistamines are given to ward off hay fever attacks. Vitamins are given to prevent deficiency states and estrogens to fend off coronary attacks in males. Local antifungal agents may be incorporated into powders for topical application to the feet as a prophylaxis against "Athlete's Foot."

Active immunity is the state of being free from contracting a particular disease either as the result of having once incurred it or being immunized against it. In either case the individual carries antibodies in his blood against the malady. Antibodies are proteins called immune globulins and they are manufactured by the body as the result of its being stimulated by a foreign substance called an antigen. This antigen may be the whole microorganism, or its breakdown products, or the toxin or poison its elaborates.

Active immunity is produced artificially by vaccines, toxin-antitoxins, and toxoids. Vaccines may contain either living or dead organisms. The Salk vaccine against polio has dead viruses, while the Sabin vaccine is comprised of live attentuated viruses. The former is injected, the latter is given by mouth. Smallpox vaccine is a live cowpox virus. Diphtheria was formerly treated with a mixture of toxin and antitoxin, but has been replaced by toxoid, which produces less reactions. A toxoid is a toxin modified chemically to yield good antibody response but not give rise to serious side reactions. Toxoids are available for immunizing against tetanus, diphtheria, and gas gangrene.

We have previously mentioned vaccines available for producing active immunity against rickettsial, bacterial, viral and fungal diseases. There is one also for the common cold, but it is actually for bacterial colds or bacterial complications of viral colds. There is no vaccine at present which will protect against all viral colds.

Allergy vaccines are used quite frequently by allergists and are directed against various allergic states such as hay fever, asthma, hives, nasal allergy, and some types of arthritis.

Passive immunity is that immunity conferred on an individual by supplying him with antibodies from another source, not from his own body as in active immunity. A newborn child received immune antibodies from its mother while in the uterus. They pass through the placenta, which is the organ that attaches the child to the womb, and enter the child's circulation. The nursing infant, in addition, receives antibodies through its mother's milk. Eventually these disappear from the child's body, when nursing ceases, and the infant then makes its own when exposed to infectious organisms. Children raised on cow's milk do not receive these additional antibodies and, after a while, lose those transmitted during their uterine existence just like the nursing infants.

Passive immunity of any type is temporary, and the body eliminates these foreign immune globulins. Serums are immune globulins. Patients who have recently recovered from an acute illness have a high antibody titre in their blood. Sometimes their convalescent serum is used to give passive immunity to others. This has been done in cases of tetanus, childhood diseases, polio, smallpox, viral pneumonias, influenza, and other illnesses. Pooled adult serums are also used so that a good mixture of antibodies will be available. These serums are known as gamma globulins, and are frequently administered to sick children who have been exposed to childhood diseases. Gamma Globulins are also injected into well children to ward off disease, and later they may receive active immunization.

Persons exposed to diphtheria, tetanus, gas gangrene, scarlet fever, and botulism (a form of food poisoning due to the botulinus organism), may be given antitoxins to neutralize the deadly toxins of the organisms causing these conditions.

Antibacterial serums are used mainly for treatment rather than prevention. They were quite widely used during the 1930's for pneumococcus pneumonia, erysipelas, and other disorders. Antibiotics obsoleted the manufacture of many antibacterial sera.

Chapter Eight

DIAGNOSTIC DRUGS

THE PURPOSE of attempting to make a diagnosis is simply to find out what is wrong with a patient. Once this is known appropriate treatment can be given. Diagnostic drugs are helpful in this quest.

In order to visualize certain organs, which are not adequately discernible on x-ray examination, it is necessary to place x-ray opaque material into them. Drugs that have this property are barium, bismuth, and iodine. Barium sulfate is administered by mouth to visualize the interior of the stomach and intestines. This preparation is insoluble and is not absorbed from the stomach or gut. It can also be given as an enema to outline the colon. Barium, in the gastrointestinal tract, helps to disclose ulcers, cancers, adhesions, strictures, diverticuli (outpockets of the colon), fecal impaction, and other types of gastrointestinal diseases.

Iodine, in either inorganic or organic compounds, is utilized for diagnosing disorders of the gall bladder and liver, kidneys, lungs, brain and spinal cord, uterus and tubes, and miscellaneous conditions. The medications may be given orally or intravenously to detect gall bladder or liver disease. The same routes can be utilized for checking the kidneys and ureters (the tubes which lead from the kidneys to the bladder). In addition, a catheter may be introduced into the bladder and then inserted into the ureters so that material can be injected to outline the ureters and kidneys. Such retrograde procedures will usually disclose obstructions, stones, cancer and other abnormalities.

Iodized oils are introduced into the bronchial tubes and allowed to trickle down into the finer filaments of the tubes and then into the alveoli, which are the terminal elements of the lungs. This procedure helps to pick up lung tumors and cancer, bronchiectasis (dilation and destruction of the bronchial walls), and emphsema (destruction of the alveoli or basic lung tissue).

To show disorders of the brain and spine several methods may be used—arterial injection, spinal fluid injection, or ventricular injection.

Arterial injections, known as angiography, are of value in diagnosing brain circulatory defects, brain tumors and cancer, brain abscesses, and arterial obstruction. The injections are made into the arteries going to the brain. Angiography is used, too, for diagnosing conditions in the heart and other organs, and also in the extremities.

Spinal fluid injections are helpful in diagnosing ruptured spinal discs, tumor or cancerous spinal cord impingements. Air or oxygen is introduced into the spinal fluid so that it will rise up and outline the ventricles (cavities of the brain) and this is known as pneumoencephalography. Any obstruction of the cerebro-spinal fluid flowing through the ventricles will be noted by this procedure and pressure upon the ventricles by tumors or cancers will be seen. Ventriculograms can be made by removing a button of bone from the skull and directly introducing a needle into the ventricles and making the injection.

Another method helpful in brain diagnosis is to inject radioisotope material which will localize selectively in a tumor or other disease process. The radioactive area is detected by radiosensitive equipment and the procedure is called brain scanning. Radioactive iodine, mercury, or technetium are the preparations now used. Radioactive isotope scanning is also utilized in diagnosing liver, thyroid, pancreas, heart, and kidney disorders.

In cases of sterility in the female, the drug is inserted in the uterus with mild pressure and, if the uterine tubes which lead from the ovaries to the uterus are open, the material will pass through into the abdominal cavity. If there is obstruction, the site will be noted. Treatment can be rendered, thus restoring patency and making conception possible.

Histamine is of value in checking stomach function. It is injected hypodermically and, in a normal stomach, will cause the secretion of hydrochloric acid. This is ascertained by putting a tube down into the stomach and withdrawing the contents periodically. When there is no free hydrochloric acid obtained, one may suspect, occasionally, pernicious anemia or stomach cancer. Quinine carbacrylic resin (Diagnex Blue®) is taken orally and the urine is tested for stomach acid secretion. This procedure obviates the passing of a stomach tube with its attendant discomfort, but laboratory technicians believe the histamine test is more accurate because of direct examination of stomach contents.

Certain dyes are used diagnostically. PSP (phenolsulfonpthtalein), a red dye, is injected hypodermically to evaluate kidney function. BSB (bromsulphalein) is injected to test liver function. Congo red is used to measure blood volume and to detect amyloidosis, a condition in which an infiltrate is deposited in many organs in chronic diseases. Sodium fluorescein, when placed in the eye, will fluoresce green at the site of an ulcer.

Endocrine substances are good diagnostic tools. Corticotropin (pituitary ACTH) may be employed for evaluating adrenal gland function. Metyrapone (Metopirone®), is utilized to investigate the hypothalmus-pituitary system. Ethinyl estradiol (Pro-duosterone®) is of value in diagnosing pregnancy. Gonadotropin yields information on ovarian function. Thyrotropin tests for thyroid activity. Insulin provides knowledge of pituitary disorders.

Glucose, a sugar, is given orally to detect diabetes and measure the severity of the disease by checking the rise in blood sugar (glucose) levels and whether or not sugar appears in the urine. Tolbutamide (Orinase®), a sugar lowering agent used in diabetes, has been found to be of value in detecting the presence of a pancreatic tumor. Another sugar, d-xylose, is employed in diagnosing a form of malabsorption, or poor absorption, of certain substances from the bowel.

Pancreatic function is judged by injecting secretin or pancreozymin. They are of value in determining the presence of obstruction, such as in tumors of the head of the pancreas where pancreatic enzyme-juices pour into the intestine. Secretin and pancreozymin stimulate pancreatic juices to flow, and, if there is obstruction, they can't get out.

The circulation time of blood flow is measured by injecting certain drugs into the vein of the arm and noting the time they are first tasted on the tongue. These observations are known as arm to tongue tests. Drugs employed for this purpose are sodium dehydrocholate, calcium gluconate, and ether. Another drug, **Fluorescite®**, after injection, will show a greenish flourescent color on the lips when observed in a dark room with a flourescent light.

An interesting drug is phentolamine (Regitine®), used to test for a rare tumor of the adrenal gland. This tumor gives rise to high blood pressure and, if its presence is established, the patient can be cured by surgery. The injection of Regitine intravenously produces a fall in blood pressure in these patients. Myasthenia Gravis, a rather rare disorder which is characterized by **extreme muscular weakness**, may be diagnosed by injecting edrophonium (Tensilon®) or neostigmine (Prostigmin®). Improvement in strength temporarily follows such injections.

Certain radioactive drugs are used in cancer detection. Radioiodinated serum-albumin is employed to localize and detect **brain tumors**. Radioactive iodine (called I^{131}) is picked up by thyroid tissue, so that one can localize spread of thyroid cancer to distant sites, by scanning procedures. Wherever there is thyroid cancer, the radioactive iodine will be present and its detection relatively easy. Radioactive phosphorus (called P^{32}) is utilized to locate tumors of the brain and eye.

Other uses have been found for radioactive materials. Radioactive chromium (Cr^{60}) is used to determine how long red blood cells live, the volume of red blood cells in the body, and fecal blood loss. Radioactive iron (Fe^{59}) is of value in determining iron turnover in the body. Radioactive cobalt (C^{60}) along with vitamin B_{12} is of value in testing for pernicious anemia. Radioactive rose bengal solution is used to determine liver function.

Some diseases may be diagnosed by certain tests performed upon the skin. The Schick test indicates whether or not a person is susceptible to diphtheria by injecting a small amount of diphtheria toxin into the skin and observing the response. If there are no antibodies to the toxin, there will be a local inflammation and the test is positive. If the person has had the disease or been immunized, antibodies will neutralize the toxin and there will be no reaction. There is a similar test for scarlet fever and it is known as the Dick test. Anyone who has been infected with the tuberculosis germ, whether having symptoms of the disease or not, will show a positive test to injected tuberculin toxin. A non-reactive test usually indicates no contact with the **organism**. Skin testing is available for diagnosing other diseases such as brucellosis, trichinosis (pork roundworm infestation), fungal infections, parasitic, bacterial, and other disorders.

Allergy skin testing is based upon the principle that allergic antibodies can be detected by applying suspected substances to the skin. This may be done by placing the material on the skin as in patch testing, by scratching the skin and putting the material on the abraded site, or it may be injected into the skin. The allergens or offending substances are manifold and consist of such diverse items as serums, foods, tree, grass, and ragweed pollens, various types of molds, dusts, bacteria, viruses, fungi, chemicals, plastics, metals, oils, detergents, soaps, paints, drugs and miscellaneous materials. If the person is sensitive to the allergen, there is a positive reaction at the site which consists of redness and an elevation of the skin known as a wheal.

It should be emphasized that diagnostic drugs testing is not necessarily innocuous. It should be known in advance whether the patient has an allergy to the medications which are going to be employed and whether or not he is a hyper-reactor to drugs. These drugs, like all drugs, may cause toxic reactions, result in exaggerated physiologic responses, produce allergic or pathologic reactions, and even kill the victim.

Recently, Robert Henkin made a most intriguing discovery. He destroyed the concept held for years that the four basic tastes are located solely on the tongue. It had been believed that salt sensation was located on the tip, sour on the sides, sweet in the middle, and bitter at the back. Henkin found that while the tongue was important in tasting, the palate, pharnyx, and larynx are also involved. By selectively anesthestizing these parts, Henkin and his co-workers discovered that sour and bitter substances are best distinguished by the palate, salt and sweet by the tongue, and that all areas of the mouth and throat show some ability to distinguish all four gustatory sensations.

Further studies showed that taste is controlled by a balance between trace metal ions such as zinc, copper, nickel and the thiols (sulfur compounds) and carbohydrate-active steroids (adrenal cortical hormones). Henkin observed that orally given doses of these trace metals to adjust an imbalance restored normal taste sensitivity. He also observed that patients with Addison's disease and cystic fibrosis of the pancreas had an increased taste sensitivity, while those with pernicious anemia and vitamin A deficiency had a decrease in taste appreciation.

Some drugs can reduce taste detection by eliminating trace metals from the body. In addition, drugs containing thiols, some used for the treatment of angina, and D-penicillamine (which causes excretion of copper and is used in Wilson's disease where there is an excessive amount of copper in the system) decrease taste acuity. Many people lose their sense of taste after an attack of the flu, but if treated with zinc regain their normal taste sensation. Research continuing in this new field with trace metals and taste awareness should prove to have much new diagnostic values.

Chapter Nine

SURGICAL DRUGS

CERTAIN DRUGS are used either before, during, or after surgery. If a patient has some condition which may jeopardize his prospects for successful surgery, an attempt will be made to correct it preoperatively. One such example is a badly anemic patient. When a patient's red blood cells are well below normal, various measures are utilized to correct the deficiency. Whole blood or a concentration of packed red cells may be given intravenously, for immediate effect. Anti-anemic drugs can also be employed such as iron, B_{12}, high potency B-Complex, folic acid, or liver concentrates if more time is available.

If the patient is generally weak, a high protein diet and supplementary vitamins are often employed. Mineral deficiencies need to be corrected. Healing and recovery are speeded up when a good nutritional status is prevalent.

If more blood than usual is expected to be lost, the surgeon will want to be sure that the blood will clot quickly. If the patient's clotting time is prolonged above normal, the surgeon will usually give vitamin K or possibly calcium. The patient's blood is typed too, in case one or more transfusions are needed.

If a patient is dehydrated, due to loss of body fluids, the body's water balance can be restored by drinking fluids. If the patient cannot take liquids orally, they may be administered intravenously. Nutrient fluids containing amino acids, sugars, and other ingredients are given by vein when deemed necessary.

Patients undergoing certain types of thyroid surgery are frequently given some form of iodine to reduce the amount of thyroid hormone in the blood. This prevents a wild, postoperative thyroid-crisis with delirium, high fever, rapid heart rate, shock and even death.

Patients with Addison's disease receive some type of steroid drug to sustain them during the critical surgical and postoperative period. These cortisone-like hormones are also ordered for individuals who have been taking these drugs for long periods of time for other conditions. Failure to provide this medication during or after surgery may precipitate a stormy period and possible death, because the body has become drug dependent for these preparations and its own adrenals are inadequate.

Preoperative medications vary somewhat with the type of surgery, and whether it is to be done under a local, spinal, or general anesthetic. Certain procedures are followed in most cases. Usually, the night before surgery, some medication is administered so that the patient will rest and get a good night's sleep. Such drugs are called hypnotics and are usually the barbiturates. Customarily ordered are products such as pentobarbital (Nembutal®), secobarbital (Seconal®), ambobarbital (Amytal®), or a combination of the latter two known as Tuinal®. Phenobarbital is seldom used anymore but is still effective. Another old time favorite is chloral hydrate.

The night before surgery, the anesthesiologist (the physician who specializes in giving anesthesia) writes certain orders. He usually prescribes the hypnotic and medication to be given in the morning just before the operation, such as an analgesic and a parasympathetic depressant. The analgesic (pain reliever) may be an opiate such as morphine, Pantopon, meperidine (Demerol®), or the synthetic pentazocine (Talwin®). In cases where deep surgical anesthesia is needed, the analgesic may be omitted. It is seldom dispensed with in local, spinal, or light general anesthesia. The parasympathetic depressant is used to block one of a dual system of nervous control known as the parasympathetic nervous system, whose activity is unwanted during surgery. The parasympathetic blocking agents prevent excessive secretions of the nasal, oral, and bronchial mucosa, thereby avoiding obstruction of the patient's airway with possible strangulation. This medication is important, especially in asthmatics and individuals with rhinitis (inflammation of the nasal mucosa), because they already have too much mucus. These drugs also relax the smooth muscle in the gastrointestinal tract, thus making abdominal surgery easier. Another effect is to dilate the pupils of the eye. Atropine, belladonna, and scopolamine are parasympathetic depressing agents. Belladonna, which means beautiful lady, derives its name from the use of the drug to dilate the pupils by Spanish ladies to create the illusion of beauty.

Anesthetics may be divided into those used for a local effect and those employed for a general effect.

Local anesthesia abolishes pain without abolishing consciousness. Drugs utilized for this purpose may be applied directly to the surface of tissues such as the skin or mucus membranes. They may also be injected into tissues of the operative site as in infiltration anesthesia, or around the nerve supplying the surgical area as in nerve block, or into the spinal region for spinal anesthesia.

Some local anesthetic drugs are used only for direct application to the skin by spraying such as ethyl chloride and Freon. Others like benzyl alcohol, amolanone (Amethone®), benzocaine (Americaine®), dibucaine (Nupercaine®), and lidocaine (Xylocaine®), are effective when applied to the skin or mucus membranes as lotions or ointments. Benzocaine lozenges have been administered for relief of sore throats. Cocaine and similar preparations are employed too, for local anesthesia of the eyes, nose, mouth, and throat.

To induce anesthesia below the skin or mucus membranes, cocaine was the initial drug tried. Because of its toxicity, other substances were gradually introduced. Procaine (Novocaine®) was among the first and is still used widely today. Also popular are lidocaine (Xylocaine®), mepivicaine (Carbocaine®), and piperocaine (Metycaine®). While relatively safe when properly used, still some individuals are subject to excessive pharmacologic, toxic, or allergic reactions when injected with local anesthetics.

General anesthetics produce unconsciousness or coma from which the patient may not be easily awakened, so that painless surgery may be performed. These agents may be administered by inhalation, rectally, or intravenously. Sometimes a combination is used, starting the patient off with intravenous anesthesia and then switching to inhalation when the individual is asleep. There are various stages in general anesthesia and they vary from light to moderate, and then deep. Extreme care must be used in the deep phase so that the individual giving the anesthetic, whether ansthesiologist or anesthetist (non-physician specialist), does not allow the patient to slip into irreversible coma and death.

Inhalation anesthesia is administered either by allowing the gas to be inhaled from a gauze mask placed over the nose and mouth or from a closed system machine with a face mask. Ether and chloroform anesthesia is accompolished by dropping the liquid on the gauze mask or even a handkerchief placed over the nose and mouth. The patient breathes in the fumes and his depth of unconsciousness depends upon the amount of anesthetic administered. With a machine, a mask is placed over the face and the anesthetic is delivered from the machine at a rate set by the person administering the anesthesia.

Diethyl Ether anesthesia, discovered in the last century, provides good emergency anesthesia or prolonged anesthesia for lengthy operations. Undesirable side effects are excitement under induction, excessive production of respiratory tract mucus, nausea and vomiting after recovery from anesthesia. Vinyl ether (Vinethane®) is used for short anesthesia only, because it may adversely effect the respiratory center in the brain, with cessation of breathing, as well as damaging the liver. Ethyl chloride and trichloroethylene (Trilene®) are toxic and therefore safe only for short anesthesia. Chloroform is seldom used in the USA due to its immediate toxic effect on the heart and its delayed action on the liver. But it is still employed in other parts of the world.

There are other gas anesthetics such as nitrous oxide and cyclopropane. The former is administered with oxygen to prevent death from lack of oxygen. It is used especially in obstetrics, because it is a light anesthetic and abolishes labor pains. It is also utilized for anesthesia induction and then the anesthesiologist or anesthetist may switch to another agent. Halothane® is a volatile liquid which produces good general anesthesia, but has toxic qualities.

Thiopental (Pentothal®) is a widely employed anesthetic and is injected intravenously. It is actually a short acting barbiturate. It can be administered as an induction agent in general surgery or obstetrical and short operative procedures, including dental extractions. It may cause respiratory depression, fall in blood pressure, and fast heart rates. Ketamine® is used like Pentothal®. However, it causes a rise in blood pressure, and probably less respiratory depression.

There are no absolutely safe local or general anesthetics. There is always a potential hazard in giving any drug which can depress the nervous system and this is exactly what they do. However, in the hands of a skilled person, there is good relative safety in case complications arise.

Previously, we mentioned parasympathetic blocking agents to relax the smooth or involuntary muscles in the abdominal organs. Deep anesthesia forces the voluntary muscles in the abdominal wall to relax, thus making the surgeon's job easier when doing abdominal surgery. However, there is a different group of drugs which can be utilized for muscular relaxation. Unlike the anesthetic agents, which act through the nervous system, they act by preventing nervous stimuli from getting into the muscle at the motor end plate, which is a specialized tissue between nerve ending and muscle.

Curare (d-tubocurarine)) and curare-like drugs (Succinylcholine® and Pancuronium®) have this property. Curare was discovered by the South American Indians who used it to paralyze their prey by placing it on their arrows. In modern surgery, the curare drugs are injected to paralyze muscles. This procedure allows for lighter anesthesia, for the anesthetic does not have to be pushed to get deep relaxation. The curare medications also are valuable in treating diseases where there are muscular convulsions such as in shock therapy, polio, tetanus, and encephalitis (brain inflammation). These drugs possess a very short action, and artificial respiration may be needed to keep breathing going, for the respiratory muscles are also paralyzed.

During the course of surgery, expected or unexpected complications may arise calling for the use of drugs. Excessive bleeding may require blood transfusions, blood plasma, fluids, or blood substitutes like dextrose. Whole blood replaces lost volume and, like plasma, adds fresh clotting factors to stop bleeding. Most bleeding is controlled by clamping and tying off of blood vessels. Pressure and tourniquets are used, too. Gelfoam and local astringents are employed to stop surface capillary bleeding. Among the latter are alum, silver nitrate, and ferric chloride. Biological agents which are normally involved in the clotting process may be used such as thrombin and thromboplastin.

Circulatory collapse or shock is the most dreaded complication of surgery. Shock is characterized by a fall in blood pressure, weak and fast pulse beat, pallid look, sweating, restlessness and confusion if the patient is conscious. When 25% of blood volume is lost by hemorrhage, shock invariably occurs. Failure to properly oxygenate the blood during anesthesia may also precipitate shock, which can be detected and corrected early by giving more oxygen. Stoppage of the heart beat, known as cardiac arrest, or respiratory failure may also be factors. Indiscrete rough handling of abdominal organs can give rise to shock. Allergic or toxic reactions to administered drugs are also shock producers.

Cardiac arrest is treated with manual massage or mechanical stimulation of the heart, while respiratory failure is treated with artificial respiration. The main symptom of circulatory failure is low blood pressure. Drugs that are of value in getting the pressure up again are epinephrine (Adrenalin®), phenylephrine (Neo-synephrine®), isoproterenol (Isuprel®), and levarterenol (Levophed®). They may be administered subcutaneously, intramuscularly, or intravenously.

Sometimes patients react adversely to drugs given just before or during the operation. Antidotes should be used where possible. Neostigmine or edrophonium will counteract curare. Antihistamines, steroids, and adrenalin neutralize allergic reactions.

Postoperative drugs are ordered by the surgeon to go into effect immediately after the operation. Pain is a most common complaint. Opiates, tranquilizers, barbiturates are given as needed. If pain is mild it may be controlled by aspirin and aspirin compounds, or Tylenol® may be prescribed for aspirin-allergic patients.

Certain drugs are used in a supporting role. During the operation blood, plasma, or fluids may be started and continued postoperatively, especially if blood or fluid loss still needs to be corrected. If, after surgery, the patient is vomiting or cannot take fluids, intravenous solutions are administered. Where certain types of stomach and intestinal operations have been performed, the surgeon may wish to rest these organs temporarily and so will give intravenous nutrients and fluids in combination. Such infusions may contain sugar and water, or saline, or balanced formulas of minerals, amino acids, and vitamins B and C.

Distress sometimes follows abdominal surgery, and the patient complains of bloating and distention. This is apt to occur following intestinal operations, due to manipulation of these organs. Gas accumulates because of this disturbance Opiates may also produce this effect. So will a lack of food in the bowels. Rectal tubes, enemas, and tubes passed into the stomach or bowels from the nose or mouth are utilized to provide relief. A drug that increases motility of the bowel and overcomes the lack of peristalsis, or sluggish intestinal movements, is neostigmine (Prostigmin®).

Another common postoperative symptom is inability to urinate. The patient feels the need to void but finds himself unable. Usually this difficulty passes without treatment. But if it does not occur, drugs like neostigmine, bethanechol (Urecholine®) or benzpyrinium (Stigmonene®) can be used to stimulate voiding. If this fails too, then a catheter can be inserted into the bladder and the urine drained off.

Vomiting can be a distressing postoperative complication Specific drugs to alleviate this condition are prochlorperazine (Compazine®), and meclizine (Bonine®), which depress the vomiting center in the brain.

Hiccuping is sometimes encountered postoperatively. It may be due to distention of the abdomen, anesthetic effects on the respiratory center of the brain or other unknown factors. Many methods have been tried to stop these spasms, but if they are all unsuccessful then drugs may be used. Breathing of carbon dioxide has been advocated. Prochlorperazine (Compazine®), promazine (Sparine®), and chlorpromazine (Thorazine®) are effective. They may be given by injection for quicker results, although they can be orally administered.

While shock may occur during surgery, it can also be a postoperative complication. Treatment is the same as previously outlined.

Heart complications may arise postoperatively from anesthesia, shock, cardiac disease, or infection. Fast or irregular cardiac rhythms, heart failure or coronary attacks may be noted. Even cardiac arrest can ensue. This calls for immediate attention, for unless heart action is restored within three to five minutes irreversible brain damage results and, if the patient survives under these conditions, he becomes a living vegetable. The medications used to combat cardiac complications will be discussed in the section under cardiovascular drugs.

Respiratory complications may also occur, resulting from anesthesia, shock, cardiac or lung disorders, or postoperative infection. If there is excessive mucus in the bronchial tubes this will have to be drained or suctioned off. Pneumonia is a common complication occurring after surgery and is treated with antibiotics. Medications employed in treating respiratory disorders will be mentioned in the proper section.

Postoperative complications involving the brain and spinal cord are occasionally seen after surgery. These may happen as the result of anesthesia, respiratory or cardiac complications, brain arterial disease, or infection. Strokes, paralyses, or other evidence of damage may be noted. Treatment for these complications call for therapy directed against the conditions causing the disorder as well as the disorder itself.

Kidney failure may be a surgical complication. This may result from anesthesia, cardiac failure, or underlying kidney disease. A complete shut down in kidney function in which no urine is formed is known as anuria. Treatment of anuria demands meticulous attention to metabolic control and sometimes the use of an artificial kidney machine to remove toxic products from the blood until the kidneys recover. In some types of spinal surgery a "cord bladder" may occur in which the bladder is paralyzed due to injury of the spinal cord.

Another complication of surgery is the formation of blood clots, especially in the blood vessels of the abdomen and legs. Long bed confinement has been shown to be a primary cause of this complication. In recent years, patients are gotten up sooner just to prevent such mishaps. The surgery itself can also be a factor in producing blood clots. In addition, some people have a tendency to blood clotting in their veins and arteries. Underlying arterial or venous disorders may also contribute to this complication.

The main danger from blood clots is their tendency to break loose in the veins and travel to the heart and lungs. This may cause death, depending of course on the size of the clot and the area it occludes. Medical treatment consists of giving anti-clotting agents such as heparin and coumarins. Surgical therapy, to stop the spread of more thrombi (clots) and their breaking loose (emboli) in the veins, is accomplished by tying off the responsible vessels. Surgical intervention may be mandatory to remove the clot from the lung if the individual's life is in jeopardy. Enzymes have been injected intravenously to try to dissolve the clots. One such promising substance is urokinase.

Chapter Ten

PSYCHIC DRUGS

PSYCHOLOGY is a word derived from two Greek words, "Psyche" meaning spirit or mind and "Logos" meaning word. Psychology is then a word or talk about the spirit or mind, hence a study of the spirit or mind. The modern psychologist has altered this definition and calls psychology a scientific study of behavior, for he claims we can never know what goes on in another human mind and measure it directly. We can only study mental happenings indirectly by what a person tells us about himself. Therefore, says the psychologist, psychology is a behavioral science, and he even goes beyond this to say it is also a biological science and a social science, even the beginnings of an applied science.

In any event, modern man is a kind of complex concoction or witch's brew—a bizarre blending of evolutionary development, genetic inheritance, environmental buffeting, and sociological pressures. His behavior must comply with acceptable standards, otherwise punishment is meted out to the transgressor.

Man's frustrations, anxieties, hostilities, and guilt feelings are all forced into a so-called normal pattern of behavioral adjustment. They may burst through this theoretical porous model into psychogenic disorders such as the neuroses and psychoses.

The subconscious mind is a storeroom of suppression and repression of both our good and bad thoughts, and the designation of good or bad depends upon the culture in which one lives. These mental cogitations are frequently of an unpleasant nature and their

Drugs, Demons, Doctors, and Disease

very presence provokes psychic turmoil and various types of complexes.

The adult male brain weighs about 3 pounds, while the female brain weighs a bit less. But when one compares the body build and stature of both sexes, the size of the brain is about the same. The human brain is exceeded in size only by that of the dolphin, elephant, and sperm whale. However, it is the ratio of the total body weight to the brain weight that matters. In this respect only the dolphin compares to man, and some claim he is superior.

The great mystery of the human brain still evades scientists. As yet they cannot tell us what constitutes memory, love, emotions, sight, hearing, and a host of other abstract and non-abstract manifestations. Some scientists despair of ever solving any of these enigmas, for they claim that the brain cannot fully define or analyze itself. For the present all we can state is what Ambrose Bierce so aptly said when he defined the brain as "an apparatus with which we think that we think."

Scientists have mapped the anatomy of the brain. The landmarks of certain physiological functions are established. We know the locations for control of voluntary movements, sensory awareness, hearing, sight, speech, emotions, smell, and other functions. But why these areas perform in this matter is unknown. Those thoughts which we are aware of in our interpersonal relations with others, and which cannot be easily reduced to mere words, has not been pinpointed. We believe intelligence is centered in the cerebral lobes of the brain, because they are the latest evolutionary development and are most highly organized in man. But in general, the brain is a vast jig-saw puzzle with many parts still missing for the final comprehension of itself. Can the brain ever understand the brain?

What is the evolutionary development of the brain? Perhaps we can learn something from this. We can watch the growth of the human embryo and see what happens. Around the fourth week of life certain patterns emerge from billions of years of progressing advancement. Fin and gill-like structures appear and then disappear. Then comes the air-breathing fish, amphibians, reptiles, and finally the primates. In the final stage the human fetus develops a tail and has hair all over the body. Before birth, these embellishments vanish. Man's brain duplicates that of its evolutionary ancestors, evolving from that of the reptile to the mammal, to the anthropoids, and finally modern man.

Anatomically speaking we have two brains—two cerebral hemispheres. Dual organs, as backup mechanisms for each other in the human body, are not unique—we have two kidneys, two lungs, two adrenals, two sex glands, even a two sided heart. The left and right brains are joined together by communicating-tract fibers called the corpus callosum. If this connection is severed by surgery, separate consciousnesses or personalities emerge. Each brain can now operate independently and perform different tasks simultaneously. In a normal human this would be impossible, for the individual would end up in complete frustration and mental collapse.

Why should there be two personalities functioning together, somehow, in the human brain? We do not know, nor do we understand, the limitations or action of the silent personality. There are more right handed people than left handed ones. In right handed individuals, the center for speech is in the left cerebral hemisphere. The left brain controls the right side of the body and the reverse is true. If the brain has its corpus callosum severed, the left brain can still speak, but the right one cannot. But it can write or motion with the left hand.

The twin personalities sleep and awaken about the same time. The individual who had this operation, and incidentally it was for relief of epilepsy, had two personalities now loose in the body, but was unperturbed by the dual phenomenon. Somehow, the personalities were compatible. The philosophical question arises now as to how many personalities are really hidden in the human brain. How many Dr. Jekylls and Mr. Hydes are struggling for ascendancy? The innumerable ghosts of the numberless individuals of the past are somehow blended with dominant and recessive traits struggling for supremacy in determining the personality at any given time.

Man is a subtle animal. When a dog barks and bares his fangs he is on the offensive. When he wags his tail he is friendly. When a man smiles and has a friendly manner, he may be ready to plunge a knife into your body. Even in a less lethal mood all men wear masks, with the exception of infants who are too young to disguise their emotions.

Humans hide their feelings and disguise their moods. We are

in fact mimics of the ancient Greek actors who wore masks to depict every temperament. The word *"Personality"* fits this performance quite well, because it is derived from the Latin "per sonare" which means "to speak through" and refers to actors speaking through their mood-depicting masks while on the stage. The psychologist uses the term "personality" when he discusses the actor, not the speaking role. Personality theories are designed to elucidate scientifically the actor along with his mask and role.

We evaluate ourselves, ordinarily, by comparing ourselves with other individuals. Is their behavior normal or abnormal? What is normal? We view normalcy as behavior which is usual or average in a culture, abnormalcy as that which differs from this accepted standard. If most people do not meet this standard at a specific time, then abnormality is the norm and what was formerly considered normal is now abnormal.

One group of people may feel that they are very well adjusted to their cultural standard, while others condemn their behavior, expressions, and thoughts as ridiculous, odd, and antisocial. What is and what is not bizarre behavior depends upon the cultural mores of a community at a definite time in history. In recent years, in our country, the standards for morality have dropped drastically with respect to sex, dress, nudity, drugs, politics, business, and social behavior. Our so-called materialistic culture defines normal and abnormal in terms of performance. An abnormal person is one who fails to perform satisfactorily in some cultural role, and is labeled accordingly. The terms "normal" and "abnormal" are useful in discussions, but are relative expressions only, and not necessarily truly factual.

Fear is universal, a gift from paleo-antiquity. Everyone has his own particular frightening thoughts. The so-called normal individual copes with his fears in a fairly satisfactory manner. The neurotic swings widely away from this adjustment to an uncomfortable compromise. He tries to hide his fears rather than abolish them, but he is still concerned that they may reappear. If he can bear this anxiety, he gets along fairly well. But if not, his behavior suffers, and this increases further his anxiety. If he can now bear this new load he will live with a fairly tense existence, otherwise a nervous breakdown may ensue.

The neurotic *does not withdraw from reality* but lives close to it, even though it is a painful world for him. He grapples with life's problems inefficiently. He experiences the same emotions as the so-called normals, but his responsive swings are much wider. He worries and is depressed more. His mental turmoil results in various body complaints, the so-called *Psychosomatic Disorders*. Among the symptoms are headache, sweating, tenseness, palpitation and skipping of the heart, nausea, stomach and intestinal pains, colitis, diarrhea, frequency of urination, muscular spasms, inability to concentrate, itching, asthma, hives, migraine, nervousness, insomnia, anxiety, restlessness. Anxiety results in a life situation of constant ups and downs.

Phobia is an irrational fear sometimes manifested in neurotics when the anxiety reaction is very severe. The individual is abnormally worried about his internal organs and their functions, heights, planes, open spaces, crowds, closed areas, germs, cleanliness, animals, and life situations.

Anxiety may drive a neurotic into an *Obsessive-Compulsion* reaction which is a persistent repetition of some thought or act. In such neurotics, obsessive fears range way beyond the normal, bringing with them severe discomfort, panic, sheer terror, and a fear of eventual insanity. They have an obsessive fear of heart disease, cancer, mental disease, or strokes. Even though told they are physically normal they cannot obliterate these thoughts. Other encountered obsessions are fear of murdering someone, sexual fantasies, repetitive words, rhymes, music, slogans, mottoes, and other trivia.

Compulsions are similar in their origin to obsessions. They also arise from the anxiety of suppressed emotions. In obsessions, the repressions are expressed in repeated thoughts, while in compulsions there is a compelling desire to repeat some physical act. The patients may continually wash their hands to get rid of germs because they are struggling with guilt feelings over sex or masturbation. They count steps, walk on cracks, strike certain objects and do other bizarre things. These people are fraught with worry and doubts about their own welfare as well as that of their loved ones.

A more primitive response is *Hysteria*, by which anxiety is eliminated or reduced by *Conversion*. The individual develops symptoms which have no organic basis and these apparently block the unconscious drives provoking the anxiety. The neurotic may temporarily lose his hearing, sight, speech, touch, as well as become paralyzed. A soldier may be paralyzed in his trigger finger because he does not want to shoot, the eye becomes blind that one may not peep, the voice is gone so that one may not speak evil.

There is also a *Dissociative Reaction* that neurotics may have. In this phase, they dissociate themselves from their conflicts by means of amnesia, which is a loss of memory, or they take on a multiple personality as in the story of *The Three Faces of Eve*. It is just another method of escape.

The neurotic, unable to cope with his problems, may go on to a *Depression*. This condition frees him from life's busy activities. He now functions at a low ebb and lives in a trough of hopelessness, fatigue, helplessness, boredom, and irritability. Sometimes depression may result from the death of a loved one. However, the depression that occurs in neurotics is much deeper and the duration much longer than in the average normal person.

Neurotic behavior occurs primarily, because of *attempts to control anxiety*, and is therefore abnormal. In *Personality disorders* we are dealing instead with people who have a *distortion of defect in their character makeup*. Everyone, of course, has some minor personality problems, for the perfect human has not yet been born. The individual with a personality disorder is severely incapacitated in his social life.

There is first of all the *Schizoid* personality. He is the shy and withdrawn person who flinches from close personal relationships with his peers. This individual does not withdraw from reality as the psychotic schizophrenic, and must not be confused with him. The Schizoid feels inadequate, inferior, and daydreams. He is often eccentric and shy. In marriage, he is emotionally frigid with both his spouse and children.

The *Cyclothymic Personality*, in contrast to the schizoid, is an outgoing extrovert who likes interpersonal relations. He swings from exhilarating to mildly depressive moods. These people have the capacity to demonstrate both warm affection and explosive anger. They mix well at work and also socially with their peers. Their moods are not severe enough to justify their being called manic-depressive psychotics. Emotional swings may occur frequently, such as every few weeks, or infrequently with years between attacks.

The *Paranoid Personality* is very suspicious of people and feels they have hostile intentions towards him. A minor degree of paranoia is common to all people. In the true paranoid personality the individual's mind is obsessed with suspicions about his fellow workers, neighbors, or family. Marital infidelity is a common suspicion. They are cold retiring people and nurse grudges. Psychiatrists believe that the paranoid personality projects on others his own personal hostilities and thoughts of infidelity which he cannot tolerate. Severe paranoid delusions are characteristic of psychotics.

There is a group of *Emotionally Unstable Personalities* who are insecure, vacillate in their moods, and cannot adjust to daily stresses and strains arising from ordinary life situations. They are undependable, excitable, and easily upset. They cannot hold jobs and make poor spouses and parents. These unstable personalities are characteristically dependent upon others, and are incapable of making their own decisions. Beneath all this helplessness are deep feelings of inferiority and inadequacy. These people are immature, selfish, demand help from others but in return offer no reciprocity and very little affection. A number of factors contribute to this type of emotional instability in childhood such as overprotection, disparagement, insecurity and rejection.

Another type of personality disorder is the *Aggressive-Depressive* individual. The *aggressive personalities* have a low fuse on self control. The normal stresses and strains of life throw them easily into fits of rage and aggression. They are dictatorial in their family life and with business associates. When everything is going fine, they can be very pleasant and charming, but if the reverse occurs there can be violent explosions. Aggressiveness is often really a false mask to hide insecurity and anxiety. Some of these personalities come from a cold, hostile background and are angry rebels when they grow up; others were given everything they wanted in childhood and are furious at the adult world for not surrendering to them. A few adopted the personalities of their brutal parents.

The *passive individual* moves to the opposite extreme and expresses little or no indignation in his interpersonal relationships, fearing that he will be disliked and shunned for any such display. Nor can he stand anyone being angry with him either, for anger is not his bag. Consequently, these people are very prone to develop anxiety, phobia and paranoid symptoms because of repressed hostilities. Due to their restrained nature they are often quite successful. For they avoid friction and are well liked. But they pay for their submissiveness by being dominated and exploited by their superiors and this treatment only deepens their resentments. Usually passive people come from families where parents have been very domineering. It is normally healthy to grumble and blow off steam at times. These people do not, and consequently suffer for their passivity.

The *Compulsive Personalities* demand meticulous orderliness in their lives. They are also very frugal and stingy, and their miserliness cools interpersonal relations with others. These people are very exacting and fastidious whether at work or at home. As executives, they demand the utmost in production, orderliness, and cleanliness. As workers they are prodigious and devoted. Housewives, with this personality, are forever compulsively arranging and cleaning their homes, neglecting their husbands and children.

Some compulsive qualities are needed in ordinary living, and are normal for everyone. Lacking these qualities completely, one would live in filth, disorganization, and disintegration. However, when compulsiveness becomes the only motivation in life, this trait becomes a complete liability. Compulsive people are devotees of the inconsequential and there is nothing else that matters in life. Work is their supreme devotion, and, if they are deprived of it on weekends or vacations, they are completely hung up and depressed. They have a guilty feeling for not being on the job. Compulsive individuals are usually very religious, very moralistic, and very conscientious.

There is another type of personality disorder, called the *Sociopath,* also known as the *Psychopath.* The terms include both antisocial people and sexual deviates. The sociopaths are fickle, cold, shallow, aggressive, antisocial rebels. Unfaithfulness is their chief characteristic. They are irresponsible in their vocations, marriages, friendships, moralities, and loyalties. Some are criminals, yet they are not astute, for they do not profit from punishment, prison, or any of their illegal experiences. The sociopaths are pathological liars and try to rationalize their antisocial and criminal acts by distorting the truth. Many are drifters too, living by their wits. Very few are successful, but if perchance they are, the sociopaths are ruthless business men or politicians. On occasion, these misfits can be very charming, but their friendships are without value, their only purpose is to use others for their own advantage.

Sociopathic development is commonly blamed on unrestricted parental catering to the child's every wish. When the youth grows up, he continues to demand his own way in everything. In childhood he missed real affection, wise discipline, and good guidance. Sociopaths are produced frequently in the slums. Ghetto children, lacking in material things, learn early to steal or go without them. Juvenile delinquents from the upper classes find there is little "action" in playing it straight. There is much more excitement and thrill in going antisocial. About 25% of the delinquents fall into the sociopathic classification; the other 75% will eventually mature, grow out of their rebellious phase, and become the square, hardworking, maligned establishment.

The Sexual Deviate is one, who is so-labeled, because he departs from publicly accepted standards of sexual behavior. Yet it is well known that many who avidly and vocally profess to uphold such standards in public, practice diverse standards privately, thereby qualifying for the title of quintessent hypocrites. According to sexologists, normal sexual behavior is whatever two consenting heterosexual individuals agree to in the privacy of their bedroom. The psychologist or psychiatrist is concerned with sexual activity only when disorders arise from the act because of guilt, and these are compulsive, destructive, anxious, bizarre, sadistic, masochistic, or other types of behavior.

The following are considered sexual deviations by current standards: Homosexuality (sex relations with one's own sex); Bestiality (sex relations with animals); Pedophilia (sex relations with children by an adult); Incest (sex relations between members of one's own family, excluding husband and wife); Fetishism (sexual satisfaction with sexual symbolic objects); Necrophilia (sexual relations with the dead).

Also considered in this classification are Fellatio (oral-sex relations with the male penis); Cunnilingus (oral-sex relations with the female genitals); Sodomy (anal-genital sex relations); Pederasty (oral-genital sexual relations between a man and boy); Voyeurism (sexual pleasure from observing people disrobe or engage in intercourse); Exhibitionism (sexual satisfaction derived from exhibiting one's sex organs); Transvestism (sexual pleasure derived from wearing the clothes of the opposite sex). Today, sex experts do not consider oral-genital or anal-genital relationships abnormal, unless they are used to the exclusion of genital intercourse.

Other deviations are Sadism (sexual satisfaction derived by inflicting pain on another) and Masochism (sexual satisfaction derived from the cruelty of a sadist). In the male, Satyriasis (excessive sexual desire) or Impotency (inability to engage in intercourse) and, in the female, Nymphomania (excessive sexual desire) and Frigidity (inability to be aroused or secure sexual gratification) are abnormal.

*It is not our purpose here to go into details of this intriguing subject. The reader is referred to our book, *Sex and the Dinosaur*, in which the subject of sex is adequately covered.

In the class of personality disorders belong the alcoholics, drug abusers and addicts. We shall comment upon them later after we discuss the psychotics.

Beyond the horizon of the anxiety-ridden neuroses and personality disorders is the land of the *Psychoses*. The inhabitants are overwhelmed with a collection of symptoms resulting from an ineffectual struggle with life. Where the neuroses leave off and the psychoses begin is like trying to differentiate between grayish-white and whitish-gray on a black-white scale. Some neuroses do become psychoses, and the question raised by psychiatrists is whether the psychoses were always there in a latent corner waiting to emerge. The venerable terms have been with us for a long time, and still serve us well as working definitions.

The psychosis represents a much wider swing away from normalcy than the neurosis. The person having this illness is in serious trouble with reality. Psychic and biologic factors in some unexplained manner produce these disorders. It may well be that genetic and biochemical irregularities supply the base from which the psychoses are created. The neurotic continues to struggle with life, whether he is emotionally beaten or not, while the psychotic retreats completely from living in his culture. Somebody once said that the neurotic lives in an unreal dream.

Psychologists claim that the non-organic psychoses are not finite diseases and have no specific causes or specific cures. Instead, they are a group of symptom-complexes indicating that the individuals, so afflicted, are wallowing about in the muddy backwaters of life, unable to meet their problems and unable to find their way out. Some authorities claim there is no such thing as mental illness in the absolute medical definition of the word "illness." They say the disorders represent, simply, unsolved problems in living, basically personality disorders. We should emphasize at this time that we are concerned with psychotics in which no organic disease can be determined, and the psychologic and social factors are clearly evident.

The psychoses are divided into three types—*Schizophrenia, Affective Reactions,* and *Organic Psychoses.*

Simple Schizophrenics are withdrawn, apathetic recluses whose contact with the world is very minimal. They usually do not have delusions or hallucinations. These people are listless and unemotional and choose an uninvolved existence.

The *Hebephrenic Schizophrenic* lives in a dream world of delusions, hallucinations, and fantasies. He may be God, Napoleon, Caesar, or any internationally prominent figure. His imaginations may take on many and varied forms.

The *Catatonic Schizophrenic* lives in a state of rigidity. He can freeze into any painful posture and hold it indefinitely with no apparent discomfort. He curtails voluntary movements and is paralyzed by an ominous fear that any activity will collapse his present rickety existence. Yet, in this immutable world, he is still subject to all types of hallucinations.

The *Paranoid Schizophrenic* trusts no one and believes other people are plotting against him. When such delusions are accentuated by mental hangups, a dangerous person may run wild, wreaking vengeance upon his supposed persecutors.

Affective Reaction individuals are manics or depressives and are usually females. About 15% of mental hospital admissions are of this type. Approximately 30% of these sufferers are *Manics.* These unfortunates are on a wild toboggan ride with an accelerating speedup. They become increasingly bewildered, raving madly while their judgement swiftly deteriorates. As the attack progresses, all aspects of the mania intensify. At the end of the attack, the patient is frequently delirious, incoherent, confused, deranged, and resistant to all attempts to bring him down. Some psychologists believe that the wild actions of the manic are really powerful efforts to fight off a latent depression. In some patients, mania and depression alternate periodically with either short or long term intervals.

The second type of affective reaction is *Depression.* In this person there is a swift decline into the deep abyss of melancholia. As the depression continues, the victim is overwhelmed by his insignificance, failures, sins, and the complete hopelessness of his life. He cannot be stimulated or cheered up, for his problems are unsolvable. He knows that no one can help him, and he considers suicide as a final solution. The patient's descent into apathy may deepen to the point where he is confined to bed and must be fed forcibly.

Another phase of this disorder may erupt into *Agitated Depression*. The depressed patient or the manic, trying to escape depression, may plunge into a state of agitated depression. The mood is melancholy, but the thermostat is set at an excited, agitated level. This drives the patient into a frenzied anxiety, with deep concern that certain catastrophic events are imminent. Consequently they reach the depths of despair in worrying about their helpless impending fate and they try to convince others of the terrible brewing crises. These fears represent chaotic thinking in the minds of the sufferers.

Organic Psychoses, in contrast to the functional psychoses we have just mentioned, have a known etiology for their appearance. Brain injuries, due to accidents, especially by automobiles, are a major cause. When brain tissue is disorganized by concussion, pressure, tears, lacerations, and actual perforations, psychoses may result.

Organic psychoses may also result from *infections* by bacteria or viruses, *abnormal metabolism,* and *poor nutrition.* Another important factor is *aging,* especially where arteriosclerosis (hardening of the arteries) gradually destroys brain tissue. The first symptoms of brain tumors may be depression. Is the brain aware of its own eventual destruction?

Another cause, which has not received the importance due it, is *allergic manifestations* of the brain and nervous system. Dohan in 1968 offered proof that some schizophrenics may be allergic. Anxiety states, migraine, paralyses, delirium, hallucinations, antisocial behavior, and other nervous system manifestations are associated with allergy.

Between 1966 and 1968, R. G. Heath, with surface and deep electric stimulation of the brain, showed that psychotic manifestations were located in the septal area of the cerebrum. He found abnormal levels of activity in brain wave recordings (electroencephalograms) coming from this area in psychotic patients. Certain psycho-mimicing drugs produced similar phenomena. Electrostimulation of the hippocampus area nearby, also produced psychotic manifestations.

Drugs, Demons, Doctors, and Disease

Heath found a blood substance, taraxein, in psychotic patients and, when this was injected into monkeys, it stimulated behavioral actions similar to psychotic manifestations. He felt it was probably the result of an allergic or autoimmune process which released histamine or a histamine-like substance. When Heath introduced histamine itself into the septal area of monkeys, they developed catatonic reactions. Psychotic-like symptoms could be produced in human schizophrenics by the drugs methionine and sulfoxamine. Heath found, too, that schizophrenics could oxidize epinephrine (Adrenalin®) faster than normals.

In addition, they have an antibody in their blood, which concentrates in the septal area to produce the psychosis. Normals do not have the antibody. This discovery implies the possibility of previous infection or other pathological involvement in the area, resulting in an allergic (auto-immune) reaction causing antibody formation.

There is a purpose in detailing these psychic disorders. Many readers have never studied psychology, and many of those who have, may have forgotten much of what they learned. The important thing to remember is that there is no such animal as a normal human being. Most of us tend to congregate around a base line called average. We all possess the seeds for developing a neurosis or behavioral disorder and pushed far enough we can go psychotic. The human brain is a labile structure which can break under enough pressure or adversity, as seen in torture and "brain washing."

The treatment of mental disorders throughout the ages is an interesting saga. The early concepts of such illnesses were that they were due to demons getting into the body. Galen, at the end of the second century, had come up with a scientific approach to the problem. He recognized the brain as being the seat of mental disorders and suggested causes such as injury, alcoholism, menstrual changes, as well as disappointment in love, shock and economic reversals. With the decline of Roman civilization, the primitive concepts again came back, namely the supernatural and magic. Demonology returned, modified by theology.

In early medieval times, mental patients were treated in the monasteries. They were given kind and humane treatment with prayers, holy ointments, holy water, the breathing on of the priests, or the application of priestly spittle, visitation to holy places, the actual touching of holy relics, even the laying on of hands. Medi-

Drugs, Demons, Doctors, and Disease

cations furnished were concoctions derived from Galen's or Hippocrates' formulations.

These mild measures, in later medieval times, were replaced by violent methods. The priests felt that laying on of hands and incantations were not sufficent to remove Satan. So they resorted to vile curses and foul epithets to drive out the devil. If the patients were very suggestible and believed in demons, such actions were successful. If unsuccessful, ecclesiastical authorities ordered the most violent methods be used to drive out demons. So torture, floggings, brandings, starvation, and anything else they could think up were visited upon the poor victims.

Later, from the 15th to the 18th centuries, mental disorders were equated with sin, especially sexual sin, and these people were considered heretics and witches. Eventually, this persecution stopped, but not before thousands of innocent people went to their death because of ignorant churchmen trying to save their souls.

The methods of treatment of mental illness in the 18th and 19th centuries have been mentioned in the chapters dealing with the history of those times. It was a conflict between violence, cruelty, and sadism on one hand and kindness, consideration, and humane treatment on the other. In the 20th century, more understanding and real advances have taken place as we shall now see.

Before treating a patient as a neurotic, one must first make sure that his symptoms are not due to some physical disorder. A general physical examination should be made. If, after this is completed, it is clearly established that one is dealing with a functional neurosis, then an attempt should be made to elicit the cause. The goal of psychotherapeutics is to give the patient a good insight into his problems and then try to change his living and environmental situations. The methods employed are determined by the individual to whom this task is entrusted be he or she a psychiatrist, psychologist, psychoanalyst, or intensive group therapist. It is not our purpose in this book to delve into this type of therapy but only to explore drug therapy in the treatment of psychic disorders.

In *Anxiety* and *Insomnia Neuroses, Sedatives* (Phenobarbital®, Butisol®, Amytal®, Seconal®, Nembutal®) have been used in the past, even in the present, but the in-drugs today are the *Minor Tranquilizers*. These ataractics or calmers are also helpful as adjunctives to major tranquilizers. Common minor tranquilizers are

Drugs, Demons, Doctors, and Disease

meprobamate (Miltown®, Equanil®), chlordiazepoxide (Librium®, and diazepan (Valium®).

Side effects of the sedatives or barbituates are drowsiness, fall in blood pressure, mental confusion, depression, occasionally addiction. Undesirable effects of Librium® are drowsiness, dizziness, confusion, headache, muscle tenderness, unsteady gait, frequency of urination. Valium's® unwanted effects are drowsiness, dizziness, double vision, hallucinations, slurred speech, headaches, incontinence of urine.

Also employed are the *Rauwolfia* drugs, which originally came from India. Prominent ones are Serpasil®, Harmonyl®, Moderil®, Raudixin®. These drugs were initially used to lower blood pressure. Rauwolfia preparations do not cause any sedation nor intensify the action of other drugs. But they increase gastrointestinal movements, slow the heart rate and dilate the pupils. Because they intensify depression, their use has declined in psychiatry.

In depressive neuroses, *Mood Elevators* such as amitriptyline (Elavil®), imipramine (Tofranil®), doxepin (Sinequan®) are prescribed.

The tension of *Obsessive-Compulsion* neuroses is relieved by Librium®, Valium®, Miltown® or Equanil®, and barbituates. Depression is relieved with Elavil®, Tofranil®, or Sinequan®.

Delirium is produced by a variety of conditions. Specific preparations given to allay this symptom are chlorpromazine (Thorazine®) thioridazine (Mellaril®), and Librium®. In alcoholics, paraldehyde is the drug of choice. Chloral hydrate calms mild agitation. Dilantin® stops convulsions.

The treatment of the psychoses made its initial advance with the introduction of chemical *Shock Therapy* in the 1930's. Insulin or Metrazole® was injected intravenously to induce shock, following which the patient went into coma. In some unknown fashion, the psychotic manifestations were relieved. Unfortunately, this was not a fully-controlled method, for the amount of drug used to produce the reaction was not exactly known, and fractures from the convulsions were a frequent complication.

Later, brain surgery came into vogue, the so-called lobectomies. In this operation, the fibers connecting the frontal lobes with the rest of the brain were severed. This operation quieted the patient but also reduced him to the status of a vegetable. Eventually, this procedure was abolished.

The next development was *Electric Shock Therapy*. It replaced chemical shock treatment, being better controlled and not as erratic. It was equally effective.

Then, in the 1950's, came the age of psychopharmacology. Tranquilizers and energizer drugs were discovered. Their application marked a new advance in treatment of mental diseases. The major tranquilizers are prescribed mainly in the psychoses, being useful in handling both acute and chronic conditions.

The *Major Tranquilizers* are the phenothiazines. Popular commercial preparations are Thorazine®, Trilafon®, Compazine®, Sinequan®, Tybatran®, Quide®, Sparine®, Mellaril®, and Stelazine®. They all have similar actions, varying only in degree. The site of their action is not fully elucidated. These drugs may affect the central nervous system, the autonomic nervous system, or both. There is some evidence that they exert a depressant action in the hypothalamic region of the brain, relaxing the psychotics and reducing their anxieties. As a result, patients are more cooperative.

Some of these drugs have additional properties which were recognized earlier than their antidepressant actions. For example, Compazine® is an excellent antiemetic (stops vomiting); Temaril® reduces itching; Phenergan® is an excellent antihistaminic. Phenothiazine side effects may include liver damage with jaundice, blood disorders, low blood pressure, symptoms of Parkinson's disease.

The main use of these medications is in treating agitated states accompanied by hyperactivity in schizophrenics, manic and paranoid states. Frequently, patients respond better to one phenothiazine than another, so that if results are not satisfactory with the initial choice, another drug should be tried.

The Antidepressants are of two types, the iminodibenzil derivatives and the monoamine oxidase inhibitors. In the first group are amitriptyline (Elavil®), nortriptyline (Avertyl®), and protriptyline (Vivactil®). Side effects are nausea, dizziness, headaches, and hypotension. The monoamino oxidase inhibitors have more serious unwanted side effects.

The monoamine enzyme system is important in metabolic processes throughout the body. Drugs which inhibit this system produce many adverse reactions, thereby limiting their usage. If the iminodibenzil medications do not work, then one can utilize cautiously the monoamine oxidase inhibitors. A frequent complication of these inhibitors is a hypertensive (high blood pressure) crisis which can have serious effects. To prevent this reaction, patients must avoid substances containing tyramine such as cheeses, bananas, chicken livers, broad beans. For, the body cannot eliminate tyramine when these drugs are taken. Alcoholic beverages, amphetamines, and concurrent administration of the iminodibenzil drugs are also dangerous when prescribing the inhibitors. Drugstore items sold over the counter may also potentiate the action of the monoamino oxidase inhibitors. Tranylcypromine (Parnate®), phenelzine (Nardil®), and isocarboxazid (Marplan®), are well known monoamine oxidase inhibitors.

While the phenothiazines have the power to induce depression, when used judiciously they may actually relieve mild to moderate cases of depression. Occasionally, the combination of a tranquilizer with a depressant may accomplish more than an antidepressant prescribed alone. This is seen in depressive patients who have mild agitation or anhedonia, where there is complete lack of experiencing any pleasure. Such a combination is Triavil® which synergizes Elavil® and Trilafon®. Other mild tranquilizers which may be used in this manner are Equanil® or Miltown®, Librium®, and Valium®.

Before the antidepressants were in vogue, combinations of amphetamines and barbituates were administered. One such compound still available is Dexamyl®, composed of dexedrine and amytal. Incidentally, it has been widely prescribed for weight reduction, the stimulating effects of the dexedrine being offset by the amytal.

Depression is one manifestation of disturbed brain circuits which may correct themselves in time. On the other hand, the disorder may knock out more circuits giving rise to a feeling of exceptional well-being or euphoria close to mania. This phenomenon is stimulated more often from electroshock than depressants.

Depression, on occasion, results in suicide. Therefore this possibility must be constantly considered and carefully evaluated. Suicide attempts occur more frequently in alcoholics, families with self-destructing tendencies, and in older people who feel that they have nothing to live for anymore.

Electroshock treatment is still indicated and used when psychotherapy has failed, suicide is probably imminent, and the psychotic depression is very severe. Such treatment offers a more rapid response than drug therapy. It is about 100% efficacious in the manic-depressive and about 80% in involutional and other depressions. Patients may relapse after electrotherapy as they do after drug therapy.

Side effects resulting from electroshock administration appear later and generally are less severe, and also disappear sooner in young patients. Older individuals get their side effects sooner, with a slower ebbing. Memory loss is the most distressing symptom and the main complaint of the patients, and this, too, eventually disappears.

There are psychiatrists like Karl Menninger, Harry Sullivan, John Perry, Julian Silverman and others who believe that certain schizophrenics will get well, will be helped by their experience, and go on to lead a more creative and constructive life. In other words their madness or craziness, and we are using lay terms now, will prove to be beneficial. Just offhand this seems wild. Most psychiatrists view the disorder in a gloomy light, something to be cleared up as quickly as possible. When this does not happen, anti-psychotic drugs are used in effective dosages.

The psychiatrists, who uphold the beneficial theory, feel that schizophrenic disarrangements are a natural reaction to severe stress in a person unable to adjust to basic life crises. Dabrowski calls this response a positive disintegration, because the psyche is trying to build and reorganize its disordered personality. Therefore any attempt to interfere with this restructuring of the mind by psychotherapy or anti-psychotic drugs is wrong because the reaction is as normal as a fever in pneumonia. This is assumed to be nature's attempt at finding a solution to the problems.

Boisen, a psychologist and chaplain, had several schizophrenic episodes himself. He feels that his illnesses were of value and that they provided a method of solving problems and thereby reorganizd his whole personality to combat personal failure and isolation. His opinion is that schizophrenic attacks either make or break an individual. One either gets well and comes out of it a better person, or failing, he becomes a pitiful wreck in a mental institution.

The question is what type of schizophrenic can make it? The answer of these psychiatrists is that the individual must have had an acute attack, lived a moderately successful life, and had some crisis just before the blowup. The chronic schizophrenic, whose

Drugs, Demons, Doctors, and Disease

symptoms have been coming on gradually over a period of time, is not likely to achieve the benefical results.

In order to understand, or better yet, to try to understand human nature, alcoholism, drug use, abuse and addiction, and those participating in rebellious and revolutionary charades, some knowledge of psychology is needed. For these reasons the subject has been briefly presented. The reader may judge for himself or herself, with a psychologic perspective, what is transpiring on our world stage and in the actors strutting about and speaking through their masks.

Let us always remember that man is molded by his inheritance, plus the pressures of environmental and sociological buffetings. There are variances in our genetic make up, but basically, in our hodge podge of genes, we have essentially the same traits. But which shall remain dominant, and which shall remain recessive, determines an individual personality. Whether we stay in the so-called normal framework of our culture or whether we slip through this fragile sieve of average normalcy into the discomforting realm of neuroses or psychoses depends upon our ability to adjust and to stabilize in an undulating world.

In looking at turbulent college students today, psychiatrist Bettelheim believes that their revolt did not actually start at the university level, but began early in childhood because of profound unhappiness and inability to fit into situations. During adolescence, these individuals begin to reject society. It is easier to attack society than to admit your troubles are due to your own shortcomings. It is a common psychological device to project one's deficiencies onto someone else, a scapegoat, in this case the establishment. These individuals nevertheless can be helped with psychiatric treatment. However some choose suicide as the way out, knowing the trouble is in their own psyche, and believing there is no solution for their problems.

All student revolutionaries are not suicide-prone. The complete antithesis of the previous type of collegian is one who attacks the university because he is unable to utilize the education it offers. He refuses to admit his own inadequacies and hates the university which is devoted to exposing ignorance and advancing knowledge. Harvard University President, Derek Bok, said that students come to the university and find what they didn't want to find; namely, that the institution cannot solve their own or society's problems.

Drugs, Demons, Doctors, and Disease

Civilized man, according to psychoanalysts, has lived on a very primitive emotional level since ancient times and this can only be upgraded by education. Present day college revolutionaries condemn education at the universities as being irrelevant, claim they have no future in a materialistic society, and therefore the entire establishment should be destroyed. They distrust our society because they claim it cannot solve world problems.

In less advanced countries people welcome our kind of technology. There is no revolt against it. In Russia the military-industrial complex is larger than that of the U.S.A, but it is not attacked by either Russian or American young people. Bettelheim feels the frustrating anxiety of youngsters is not the Vietnam war or the nuclear bomb, but the belief that American technology has passed them by. Most rebellious students are from middle-class, affluent families. Too little responsibility and too much materialism and permissiveness have given them too much free time to stir up trouble. Many intelligent students, despite their thinking, are actually immature and act like spoiled children having temper tantrums, striking down straw men to relieve their frustrations. Instead of facing reality, many young people cop out. They flee into hippie and drug cultures, exotic and mystique religions and philosophies.

When America was not affluent years ago, and most youngsters could not go to college, there were little opportunities for revolt. The young had to go to work and were not supported by their parents. Today there is a choice, college or work. Some of those who choose college revile our so-called society and refuse to pursue what they term are valueless goals. Being financially dependent on their folks frustrates them and so they hate their parents. They dislike all authority, a carry-over from childhood. Pent up hostility is vented against the establishment which is symbolical of their parents. This nonsensical thinking is positively valid in their immature psyches, and so protests, destruction, violence and revolt against society is fully justified.

In all societies there must be controls, lest they sink into chaos. Freud calls this anarchy barbarism and says it is barbaric to destroy savagely. Yet even barbarians have a code for themselves. Primate societies, too, have some organized structure, especially the chimps, monkeys and baboons. This new wave of atavistic barbarism, says Bettelheim, must be combatted by allowing only those students to enter college who have the ability, interest, and desire to pursue

Drugs, Demons, Doctors, and Disease

vigorously a college education. The others should be allowed to enter non-collegiate professions, trades, and services. In this way they can be active and feel needed, thus negating their complaint that they are unwanted and rejected. Bettelheim also suggested that a youth service program be set up for the young to provide work with payment. After this service is completed, those who sincerely want to go to college would be admitted.

The universities have been under heavy pressure to provide more education in recent years. Excessively large student enrollments have only resulted in increasing impersonal student-faculty relationships, and so students feel like nameless imprints in an inhuman computer. The criticism has been leveled that the university has not kept pace with the times, and there is merit in this judgement. Immature students are disenchanted and want the university to change the curricula to meet their own deficiencies. In trying to meet all the demands, both rational and irrational, the universities are in an agonizing dilemma. Therefore some students cop out, others wait for a Godot who never comes, while others follow the piping of the Pied Pipers of militancy.

In trying to appraise these problems, Wendell Johnson believes that people bring on their own emotional problems by concentrating on their unrealistic ideas of life, and that these misconstrued opinions carry their own in-built frustrations, upheavals, and strains. If one cannot fill the void in his life with meaningful activities, an apathy sets in which gives rise to impotence, addiction, and self-destructive hostility.

J. Barzum, in the symposium "Man and Life," searching for answers, asks the question, "Is life worth living?" This question can only be answered on a personal basis, and many are answering "no." Barzum attempts to analyze the reasons which have caused deterioration of the quality of life. The first reason is the complaint of impersonal encounters with others. This causes a breakdown in manners and a feeling of alienation, of being manipulated like a cog in a machine. Such attitudes lead college students to reject the university curricula as lacking relevance, and they are frustrated by being educated for a society they distrust and dislike.

Secondly, Barzum notes the failure to get things done that need to be done. There is, consequently, a lack of satisfaction for real accomplishment. Thirdly, Democracy is a factor, for it emphasizes the drive for equality which sparks envy and competition. This in turn calls for self-examination that can lead to depression. Because of stress on equality, the hero is gone and the anti-hero is the man of the day. Strong leadership is missing because ambition and power are distrusted. There are no more great causes. We are at the end of an era.

DRUG USE, ABUSE, AND ADDICTION

Now that we have some ideas of why people act, think, and do as they do, let us go to the important subject of drug use, abuse and addiction.

A physicians' panel, testifying before a Senate subcommittee, blamed advertisers for inducing individuals to take too many drugs. The doctors claimed that advertisements were persuading the public not to accept minor discomforts. People are coaxed to pop pills for fast relief, pleasure, freedom, comfort, sleep, relaxation, and regularity. The consumer is constantly bombarded to take medications. Consequently our young people accept this misinformation as truth and use drugs to cure or solve their problems, real or imagined. As many of the advertisements do not live up to their Madison Avenue mirages, people consult their physicians looking for the promised land in miracle medications.

Life in our times is at best quite difficult, with problems in family life, business, society, politics and the domestic and foreign scenes becoming more complex all the time. The stresses and strains reflect themselves continuously in our daily living. Consequently, people like to reduce their physical and mental annoyances to a minimum. Hence there arises the urge to take medicines, aided and abetted of course by the huge advertising campaigns on TV, radio, magazines, newspapers, and other media. For many people medicines become a crutch for daily living. Use frequently becomes an over-use or abuse. With some drugs abuse leads to addiction.

The universal cry is for an escape—to get away from the rat race. "Stop the world I want to get off" was a common expression a few years ago. As this feat is impossible, one must live here on earth with one's anxieties, frustrations, fears, pains and aches.

Huge quantities of mild pain relievers (analgesics), in which aspirin or aspirin-like ingredients are present, are consumed every day. Among these are plain acetylsalicylic acid (aspirin), salicylates, slow release aspirin such as Measurin® or Persistin®, Tylenol® (acetaminophen), Darvon® (dextropropoxyphene), Empirin®, phenacetin, aminopyrine, and acetanilid. The last three medications are used very seldom now because of the possibility of adverse reactions.

Tranquilizers, sedatives, and hypnotics are widely prescribed and consumed in large quantities by the public. A vast proportion of our population depends upon these medications for their daily mental and physical sustenance. They believe that they cannot get about, do their chores, keep on the job, keep their nerves quiet and sleep, unless they have drug help. Of course there are sound medical reasons why some people need these drugs on a temporary basis, and even some on a permanent basis, but in general there is over-use or abuse of these preparations. Our psychologic perspective should have made it clear by now why drugs become crutches for a large proportion of our present day society. Drugs of the type we are discussing do not solve problems, they make them less audible and visual.

While addiction may take many forms and involve various medications such as sedatives, tranquilizers, and hypnotics, the most serious problems of addiction are concerned with nicotine, alcohol, opium and its derivatives such as morphine, heroin and demerol, along with marihuana, and amphetamines.

SMOKING

Smoking is generally considered a habit, but to many smokers it is nicotine addiction. If they try to stop they get withdrawal symptoms of headaches, nausea, and extreme nervousness with a craving "to grab a smoke." Cigarette smoking usually begins in adolescence, as youngsters try to ape their elders and conform to the habits of their peers. There is also a feeling of being more adult and more mature by this habit.

Smoking provides a variety of satisfactions. It gives the individual something to do. It allays nervousness and relaxes the individual when tense or upset. There is also the psychological pleasure of watching the curling of the smoke, which a blind person cannot see and so he does not enjoy smoking. According to psychoanalysts, cigarettes act as "oral pacifiers," providing temporary relief from daily tensions and strains of living. Compulsive smoking, in some cases, is said to be a masochistic drive to self destruction.

The hazards of smoking are well known: bronchitis, emphysema, lung, mouth, and throat cancer, heart and blood vessel diseases, reduction of life expectancy.

For the person who has given up smoking, the greatest urge to go back to the habit is at the cocktail hour. Pharmacologist Budh Bhagat believes this is due to the combined effect of nicotine and alcohol on the production of the hormone norepinephrine, also called noradrenalin, which is utilized in maintaining blood pressure, blood sugar and metabolic rate. In the brain, it helps to maintain emotional balance. Using rat experiments, Bhagat noted an increase in production of the hormone after ingesting alcohol, but persistent drinking causes a breakdown of the noradrenalin and a sharp drop in its presence in the blood, accompanied by anxiety and depression. On the other hand, nicotine increases production of the hormone and also its use in brain metabolism. As alcohol decreases the norepinephrine level, the urge to light up a cigarette and increase the norepinephrine levels again becomes almost irrestible.

Robert Elliot noted that red cells of smokers have a reduced ability to carry oxygen, which is not due to carbon monoxide in the smoke. This is equivalent to about 20% of the blood being pumped around and not transporting oxygen. Since the heart has a high oxygen requirement, this oxygen deficiency may account for the increased risk of heart muscle damage and coronary thrombosis. Carbon monoxide has a damaging effect on the heart muscle, also the conducting system of the heart.

Smoking is associated with sudden deaths from coronary disease. David Spain noted that sudden deaths in heavy smokers were 16 times more frequent than in non-smokers. Thirty percent of non-smokers survived more than an hour but only 5% of heavy smokers. There is a low prevalence of coronary thrombi or clots in cases of sudden death, thrombi being probably a secondary and not a primary event. Paul Astrop and other Danish scientists note that carbon monoxide make the walls of blood vessels more permeable thereby allowing cholesterol and other fats to clog vital arteries. They feel that we should be concerned with all forms of carbon monoxide exposure today, not only that from smoking.

How do you get people to stop smoking? The answer is you can't, unless they really want help. The tenacity of the smoking habit is a real challenge to behavioral psychologists. If we can't control this "simple problem," they say, how can we hope to be effective against alcoholism and drug abuse. Anti-smoking drugs are not too efficacious. There is available both individual and group therapy to combat smoking. There is also the cold turkey treatment, in which one goes off smoking completely; the other method is the slow reduction of the number of cigarettes consumed daily. Unless the motivation to quit is strong in the individual, he will relapse. Today we have many successful people who have kicked the habit, and we also have many who tried and never quite made it.

ALCOHOL

Alcoholism is reputed to be as old as the human race. It may be defined as the compulsive drinking of alcoholic liquors. Just when primitive man found that fermented grains yielded an exhilarating high, is not and may never be known. There are, of course, occasional and chronic drinkers. The sporadic imbiber can hardly be called an alcoholic. The habitual consumer is an alcoholic.

John Tamerin and associates of the National Institute of Health state that alcoholics drink not to feel better and be more sociable, although this seems to be a conscious rationalization, but rather to regress into the past, rebel, and to bring forth and act out impulses and wishes repressed from their early lives.

Alcoholism is a familial disease. Male relatives of the alcoholic have a high risk for alcoholism, while female relatives show a strong affinity for affective mental disorders, according to psychiatrist George Winokur and his associates. In a group of alcoholics studied by this group, the family history demonstrated noticeable evidence of mental illness and psychiatric symptoms. The alcoholics themselves showed definite mental disturbances, with a decline in their general and mental health.

Psychiatrist Morris Chafetz of Boston observed that children of alcoholics had an above average risk for developing alcoholism, and were more apt to suffer emotional disturbances and deviate behavior than were children of non-alcoholics.

It is probably a myth, says Chafetz, that recovered alcoholics can't be social drinkers. He doesn't know for sure. He thinks that insistence on complete abstinence may not be the ideal objective for these people, because they may develop anxieties, ulcers, and lose their associates. How valid this thinking is, is questionable. It may possibly apply to a small few, if at all. Is an alcoholic ever completely recovered? The answer seems to be no.

Chafetz insists on seeing and treating the whole individual in his total social system. Eleanor Clark of the Massachusetts General Hospital, working under the psychiatrist's supervision, reports excellent results in helping these unfortunates with group therapy. Motivation must be first established along with ego building. This stimulation can be created in an association with their peers in group therapy, which acts as a substitute family and a small community in which they all have the same problems. In this environment, they help one another and many return to a useful life in their city.

The results of alcoholism are pretty well known. Long continued use may result in nutritional disease (from lack of proper eating), cirrhosis of the liver, mental disorders and insanity, increased susceptibility to infection, inefficiency on the job, accident proneness, automobile accidents. Recently, Gould and Comprecht of Misericordia-Fordham Hospital of New York showed that alcohol directly damages the heart and that cardiac damage is not necessarily secondary to cirrhosis of the liver.

The most publicized complication of alcoholism is cirrhosis of the liver. G. A. Martini of West Germany states that there is virtually no cirrhotic who drinks less than 80 Gms (3 ounces) of alcohol a day. He also claims that 80% of cirrhotic cases in France are due to alcoholism. The liver is often referred to as the most overworked, underrated and abused body organ. It performs over 500 functions. One of its most important actions, outside of participating in general metabolism, is to destroy and neutralize harmful substances such as chemicals, excess histamine, drugs, poisons, and toxins of bacterial fungal and viral origins. Alcohol interferes with this function.

In 1968, the Supreme Court of the United States ruled that alcoholism is not a disease but rather a paralysis of will power. To convince the judge, the alcoholic, and the physician, that alcoholism is an addictive disease, positive evidence must be demonstrated. Virginia Davis and Michael Walsh, biochemists of Baylor College of Medicine, determined to find it. A theory advocated in 1968 suggested the initial oxidized metabolite or chemical spinoff of alcohol is acetaldehyde, and this substance along with noradrenalin produces a morphine-type drug (of the tetrahydroisoquinoline family) in the body. A newer theory in 1970 suggests that alcohol may indirectly interfere with the chemistry of the brain to produce another morphine-type drug of the same chemical family.

Davis and Walsh believe that the whole basis of alcoholic addiction is altered dopamine (which is the brain chemical lacking in Parkinson's disease). This change is brought about by alcohol and acetaldehyde. According to these biochemists, then, alcoholics are not addicted to alcohol but to an addicting substance created in their bodies by drinking alcohol. The doctors experimented with rats and found that, in the normal process of oxidation, metabolites of dopamine and alcohol compete for an enzyme (aldehyde dehydrogenase).

Because there is more of the aldehyde of alcohol present to react with the enzyme, than that of the dopamine, the excess of the latter's aldehyde is converted to another substance known as THP (a tetrahydroisoquinoline substance) which is the same substance found in the opium poppy before it becomes morphine. These investigators believe that THP is then converted into an addicting drug. Therefore one must conclude that alcoholics and drug addicts are similarly afflicted. Now that we have finally gotten some biochemical facts on what causes alcoholism, perhaps an antidote may be found eventually.

A common disorder of drinking is the well known "hangover." According to neurologist Donald Dalessio, fifty million Americans drink alcoholic beverages. A large proportion have experienced hangovers, which, besides being distressing, cause loss of time and income in business. New studies are throwing light on this distressing disability.

What are the effects of alcohol and how do they cause hangovers? Dalessio points out that alcohol first dilates or opens up blood vessels. Faces flush. This rosy glow is first noted in the blood vessels of the skin. The drinker at this time exhibits a sense of well being, warmth and good fellowship to his fellow imbibers. Alcohol further increases the ruddy glow by speeding up the heart, increasing blood pressure and pulse rate.

Alcohol probably acts directly on the brain centers which control blood vessels and heat formation. It also affects areas concerned with emotions, thereby producing a feeling of calmness and tranquility, which is the main reason for its ingestion initially. Then follows the usual loosening up of the individual who now becomes party conscious with laughter and singing, and carrying on with acting, dancing and profuse talk.

Alcohol causes an increase in urine output which is apparent to all drinkers. This diuresis is produced by direct action of alcohol on the brain which incites a brain hormone to stimulate the kidneys. More urine is excreted than fluid is taken in as a rule. The heavy imbiber soon finds himself dehydrated.

The drinker rarely consumes pure alcohol which is odorless and colorless. Instead, he drinks liquors which contain alcohol, water, and congeners which give them color, aroma, taste, and flavor. These congeners may come into the distillant directly from the grains used, or else indirectly from the storage containers such as vats. The congeners are composed of varying amounts of such substances as acetic acid, furfural, fusel oil, tannins, aldehydes, various esters and unknown substances. They may exert a toxic action of their own.

We may now analyze the hangover more fully. The severe headache accompanying the condition is due to overdilated blood vessels which cause the intense throbbing, synchronous with the rapid heart beat. The headaches is aggravated by moving, changing position, or any polting. Nausea or vomiting may occur because alcohol stimulates the vomiting center of the brain. The severe headaches can also cause gastric discomfort, while nausea may reflexly aggravate the headache. The overworked liver may also vent its displeasure. Dehydration adds to the nausea, and a desire to drink, to allay thirst, brings repercussions from an angry stomach.

The drinker, at this time, is in an irritated state, because his brain has had it between the booze and the overactivity from the night before. All noise becomes absolutely unbearable. The fatigued brain is looking for peace and quiet.

How can we successfully treat the hangover? Since the overdilation of the blood vessels is a prime cause of discomfort, a constrictor is needed. Ergot derivatives such as ergotamine, used in migraine, are helpful. Caffeine, present in coffee, also works. Some preparations are available which contain both drugs. If the person cannot hold anything on his stomach these medications can be taken as rectal suppositories. An ice bag to the head gives relief. Antihistamines are both antiemetic (antivomiting) and sedative.

Dehydration can be overcome by supplying fluids such as broths, which are salted, because the body needs salt and water. Blood sugar is usually low, and, if the nausea is not too severe, orange juice can be taken to raise the level. Lowenstein and coworkers of Boston University and Harvard medical schools discovered that the sugar fructose was the most effective agent for increasing the metabolism of alcohol and getting the patient out of his dilemma more quickly. Fructose is present in honey, ripe fruits, vegetables and their extracts. A common source of this sugar is tomato juice, which has been advocated for years as a "morning after drink" for hangovers. This advice we now see is based upon good scientific facts.

To prevent hangover, it has been suggested that one consume toast spread thickly with honey before retiring after a night of heavy drinking. Drinking of vegetable juices, too, will also be beneficial in metabolizing the alcohol. They can also be served in the morning especially the favorite tomato-juice cocktail.

Dalessio astutely notes that ingestion of pure alcohol produces far fewer symptoms than the drinking of alcoholic liquors. He suggests that pure alcohol would be preferable for drinking. Of course the price is very high due to governmental taxation. He furthermore states that vodka is the purest of the liquors available and contains the least amount of congeners. Of course, the only absolute preventative against hangovers is not to drink. To expect this of our present culture is to expect the impossible.

Pychologist David McClelland says we have to search for the reasons behind the reasons men give for doing what they do. His own personal quest resulted in several disclosures. One he calls "n-Ach," the *need* for *achievement*. Later he discovered the *need for power* while investigating why people drink. This led to the *need for affiliation* which some call the love motive.

In an article on the "Power of Positive Drinking," McClelland states that studies on alcohol have been biased by the Prohibitionist idea that it is a drug with bad effects, biased by the failure of psychologists to concoct joy in the laboratory, and finally biased by the American credo that action alone is substantial and real, while fantasy is not. He claims his studies provided no proof that drinking is an oral gratification or dependent fantasy as alleged by psychiatrists. Anxiety fantasies did not decrease after a few drinks. What did increase were thoughts of power—power of impact on others, power of aggression and sexual power.

Later McClelland was able to discern two types of power—p-Power (personal dominance over others), or s-Power (power to be used to help others). At cocktail parties he noted that, after 2 or 3 drinks s-Power thoughts predominate. After heavy drinking fear and anxiety decrease. As one becomes less inhibited p-Power takes over.

The heavy drinkers is the man with excessive desire for personal power. Drinking fuels this need. The power-drunk mood calls for more drinking, intoxication, fighting, accidents, marital discord and sexual exploits. David Winter noted that heavy drinking collegians found their power outlet in sexual conquests and high-powered cars or motorcycles. Those individuals with s-Power, whether collegians or workers, serve in voluntary social organizations.

What is this mania for power? There are many factors. In our society the responsibilities of men increase, through middle age, while their physical capacities decrease. Accordingly, men of this age drink more than younger men.

Psychologist Robert Goldenson, in his *Encyclopedia of Human Behavior,* claims that there were 70 million users of alcohol in the USA in 1970 with 5 million alcoholics and 200,000 being added each year. Alcoholism is the 4th most prevalent disease in the country, accounts for 15% of admissions to mental hospitals and is a leading cause of death. It costs 1.25 billion dollars a year to care for, treat and support these people and their families. A large percentage of arrests and 15% of murders are caused by drinking. Eighty percent of drunkards are men and only 5% are skid row bums, the rest come from the middle and upper classes. The life span is reduced by 12 years for alcoholics. The majority of automobile accidents are caused by drinking drivers, killing 30,000 people a year. These statements are very impressive and are a serious indictment of an alcoholic culture.

Goldenson characterizes alcoholics as immature, passive-dependent persons, who try to achieve unrealistic goals. They cannot tolerate anxiety, failure, criticism, or tension. They drink to bolster confidence, appease their maladjustments, relieve loneliness, eradicate inhibitions, and anesthetize feelings of futility.

He suggests that acute intoxication be treated in the hospital, with tranquilizers being used to relieve nausea, induce sleep and prevent withdrawal symptoms. The drug Antabuse® can be tried to prevent future drinking. If the patient is given Antabuse® and then drinks alcohol, he becomes very sick. This sets up a condition reflex which may make the individual forsake liquor. Psycho and social therapy are suggested for giving the patient an insight into his problem and enabling him to adjust his life more satisfactorily.

In conclusion, it can be seen that the drinking of alcohol is viewed differently by various authorities. Their personal preference for, or distaste of alcohol, colors their expressiveness. So both standpoints are prejudiced. Taking a middle of the road course, and noting the statistics of Goldenson and other sources, one can only conclude that alcoholism is a tragedy of the highest magnitude and a travesty on our culture. As bitter as this calamity is, it is perhaps no worse than any other drug addiction. The difference is that it is acceptable by our society and is legal.

SEARCH FOR THE HIGH—FLIGHT FROM REALITY

Reality is the state of things as they are, unreality is the state of things as we wish they were. Reality is harsh, fearful, uncomfortable, painful. Reality is suffering, sorrow, servitude, sickness, shallowness, suicide; reality is defeat, destruction, deceit, disappointment, depression and death.

Reality is ourself, other people, and nature. At times, it is quite difficult to live with oneself, because of the problems and mistakes we bring upon ourself. It is even more agonizing to tolerate and get along with others, for we love and are more forgiving to our own ego. The hardships brought upon us by an indifferent and uncompromising nature are most frustrating. It is difficult to achieve peace and serenity for ourselves in this world.

Everyone seeks to escape from the continual blows of the three components of reality—ourself, others, and nature. Some have turned to monotheistic or polytheistic religions, mysticisms, and the occult. Others seek brief periods of evasion in pursuits such as books, movies, radio, TV, the theatre, athletics, hobbies and sex. Still others have tried to compensate by pursuing success in business, religion, arts, and the professions. Then there is the turned-on world of drugs.

Norman Taylor, in his book *Narcotics: Nature's Dangerous Gifts*, when speaking of the flight from reality, says that men have always wanted that help which religion and philosophy have never given them. What men actually want is some brief respite from the disillusionment of reality, not the oblivion of a mystical or hypothetical heaven from which there is no return. They want a little bit of heaven right here on earth. Soviet politician Krushchev echoed this thinking when he said that religion offers the workingman pie in the sky, but communism supplies it right here on earth.

Everyone seeks to escape from the constant buffeting of actuality. The immediate problem for all of us it how can we flee our present existence. Everybody wants to be happy, to achieve the *HIGH* which takes them into new realms of joy, delight and forgetfulness. How can we attain Nirvana?

Some experience it temporarily in the hot swirling smoke of the cigarette or the pleasant feeling of the warm tingling cocktail. Ancient man not only discovered alcohol, but he also discovered drugs by which he could soar to new heights of tranquility and peace, where pain and boredom did not exist.

Man has sought for and gained *HIGH* in many ways. One has been religion and mysticism. St. Augustine tells of a mysterious force which seized and carried him off into a wonderous world of dazzling lights and indescribable joy. He passed beyond rational intellect and called this force God. St. Teresa told of supernatural ecstacies in a world of transcendental light and wondrous bliss, and where instantaneous knowledge was acquired. St. Paul saw a blinding light and heard the voice of Jesus on the road of Damascus. Peter, James, and John saw Jesus in a dazzling whiteness at the transfiguration, and from a cloud came the voice of God.

Ramakrishma, Indian mystic, envisioned a shining ocean and an endless enchantment. From all sides gleaming waves engulfed him and he knew no more. God, he said, is in everything and everything is God.

Carl Gustav Jung, famous psychiatrist, said that he had encountered shattering experiences with the Lord in his dreams and visions, similar to those of oriental mystics. He felt that there was no inner peace for Carl Jung until he had plunged into the depths of his own mind and discovered himself. At every step he found the psychic material of which psychoses are made and which confuse the mental patient.

Ancient man looked for a high and an escape from his harsh existence. By experimenting, he gradually found that he could gain this objective by using opium, marihuana, peyote, mescaline and other botanical materials.

In the 19th century, James Simpson gave one of the first chloroform parties. A young lady, under the influence of the drug, cried out that she was an angel and was beginning to fly. A naval officer began to crow like a cock. The staid Simpson stood on his head. When he recovered, he declared that chloroform was better than ether, indicating that he had tried that too. This man was the great Scottish obstetrician who introduced chloroform anesthesia for childbirth.

Sir Humphrey Davis, in 1798, experimented on himself with nitrous oxide gas. He discovered thrilling sensations in which objects became dazzling to look at and sounds were deafening. He floated in a world of new ideas and objects. He suggested the use of this gas in surgery.

Crawford Long, in the last century, indulged with friends in ether parties and became unconscious. Later he applied this knowledge for surgical anesthesia.

Seturner, in the 19th century, isolated morphine from opium. Its wonderful dreamlike producing effect, and its ability to kill pain, stimulated the inventor to call it morphium in honor of Morpheus, god of dreams and sleep. It, like opium, is an addicting drug.

Cocaine brought similar habituating hazards to its experimenters. Sigmund Freud took it and suggested it as a cure for morphine addiction. He found, in using it on himself, that cocaine lifted him out of his depressions into an exhilarating state and the euphoria he then enjoyed was similar to one being in excellent health. As soon as he detected the dangers of addiction to cocaine, he discontinued using it.

At the end of the nineteenth century, investigators in the USA and abroad wore distorting lenses of various types to confuse their visual interpretations of the world. They saw bizarre shapes, contortions, color mixtures. After a few days, the brain was able to decipher the situations and the unreal world became real again.

Aldous Huxley, Havelock Ellis, and others tried peyote and mescal. Silas Weir Mitchell smoked hashish and wrote about its effects. In 1896 he sent some to the philosopher William James, saying he had been in fairyland under its influence. James, however, got violently ill after trying it.

The Swiss biochemist Albert Hoffman accidently took lysergic acid in 1943. This serendipitous act precipitated a massive self-use and experimentation with hallucinogenic drugs.

A present day counterpart to the experimenter Weir Mitchell is psychiatrist Humphrey Osmond, who is one of the outstanding pioneers on model psychoses. He is the man who coined the word "psychedelic." Osmond has described his personal experiences with many drugs, a few of which are peyote, LSD, mescalin, psilocybin, dimethyltryptamine, and morning glory seeds.

MARIHUANA ("POT")

The earliest description of the use of marihuana is in a pharmacy book written about 2737 B.C. by the Chinese emperor Shen Nung. Even then there was strong opposition to the drug. From China the use of the hemp plant spread to India, then to North Africa, and finally Europe.

Scientifically the plant is known as Cannabis Sativa. It grows as a common weed in many parts of the world including the USA. There are both male and female plants. It is from the latter plant that one gets the sticky marihuana resin which is extracted from the flower clusters and the top leaves when the plant is ripe.

The hemp plant has been employed as a source of fiber for making rope, textiles, birdseed, as an intoxicating drug for tribal religious ceremonies and as a medication. In the 19th century, marihuana was prescribed in the USA for coughs, asthma, pain, rheumatism, migraine and other headaches, insomnia, anxiety and exhaustion. The name marihuana is believed by some to be derived from the Portuguese word "mariguango" meaning intoxicant. Others say it is a Mexican-Spanish name. The product was outlawed in the USA in 1937.

The drug is produced in several different grades and these are called by their Hindu names, for the Indians were experts in cultivating and preparing the extracts. The poorest and cheapest grade is known as bhang. It is derived from the cut tops of non-cultivated plants and is low in resin content. This is the type smoked chiefly in the USA, despised by the Hindu connoisseur, and used only by the very poor Hindus.

The next higher grade is called Ganja, and is derived from the flowering tops and leaves of cultivated plants, thereby producing a better quality and quantity of resin. The highest and best quality preparation is known as charas or hashish. This is made only from resin which is scrupulously removed from the tops of mature cultivated plants.

The chemistry of Cannabis sativa is very complex and the chief ingredients are believed to be isomers or close relatives of the chemical called THC (tetrahydrocannabinol). Recently one of these has been synthesized and called delta-1 form. It is assumed to be the main substance giving the high from the plant. Marihuana is usually smoked, but may be baked into cookies and candy, or mixed with honey for drinking or prepared as a tea.

Psychiatrist Walter Bromberg of New York in 1934, after an extensive study of marihuana, described the psychic effects of the drugs after observing and talking to users. His description is classical.

He says that, about 10 to 30 minutes after smoking, the user encounters an anxiety period associated with restlessness and hyperactivity. This episode disappears shortly and is replaced with calmness followed by euphoria, talkativeness, exhilaration, and feelings of lightness of the body and extremities. The individual laughs explosively and uncontrollably for no apparent reasons, believes he is very witty and a brilliant conversationalist.

The marihuana smoker's processes then begin to speed up. He may now experience visual hallucinations and see brilliant lights and colors which coalesce to form various shapes, faces, designs and complex configurations. There is a dulling of time and space perceptions. Eventually he falls asleep, and, when he awakens, there are no physiologic after-effects. Memory is usually clear for what transpired during marihuana intoxication. Most observers confirm this description as a good composite picture of marihuana highs. Effects of smoking last for 2 to 4 hours, while the effects from ingestion of the drug last for 5 to 12 hours.

A new user of cannabis may have an initial period of anxiety which frightens and panics him. His friends will usually comfort him and talk him down from this high. Experienced indulgers label this a happy high. They also claim that it gives them an appreciation of music and art which would not be ordinarily available in the non-high state. Many musicians contend that their performance is accentuated under the influence of marihuana. Some smokers state that there is a kind of dualness under the high, one personality being intoxicated and the other laughs or ridicules it. Marihuana differs from other hallucinogenic drugs in that it is less potent and still produces the same effects.

A recent report by the British Public Health states that marihuana produces a rapid pulse rate, fast shallow breathing, tremors of the tongue and mouth, red eyes and an unsteady gait. Physicians at the Boston Veterans Hospital stated that six patients who injected marihuana in their veins developed fever, fast heart rate, vomiting, diarrhea, drop in blood pressure, kidney failure and blood alterations. Zinberg and Weil, in their study, said that the heart rate was increased and the eyes reddened, but contrary to common belief, the *pupils of the eyes were not dilated.*

First time smokers do not get euphoric highs, the latter must be learned. Edward Truitt, Jr. suggests that THC is converted to an active substance by liver enzymes which increase with repeated drug usage. This may explain why beginners are unaffected until the marihuana is utilized several times.

Stanford University researchers reported that large oral doses produce disorganization with relation to speech, thinking and time. Weil and Zinberg found little difference psychologically between moderate and nonusers in a group of collegians, but chronic users demonstrated intellectual deterioration, antisocial attitudes, extreme anxiety and a vague paranoia. Former army psychiatrists, Talbott and Teague, reported frequent and severe adverse reaction in American soldiers in Vietnam where marihuana is very potent and cheap.

Psychiatrist Lester Grinspoon of Harvard University, in summarizing the activity of marihuana, says it is a mild intoxicant, it is not addictive, does not incite criminal conduct nor does it lead to physical or mental degeneracy. Chronic heavy use, as in the Orient and Middle East, may lead to debilitation just like the heavy chronic use of alcohol. He astutely raises the question as to whether these heavy smokers and ingesters were not already hopeless and defeated people before starting the drug. Which comes first, the personality disorder or the drug? It's the old story of the chicken and the egg and which comes first. Grinspoon applies this same question to the "potheads" of today in the USA. Many of these college students had conflicts and depressions before starting marihuana.

In critically comparing the effects of alcohol and marihuana, the

Drugs, Demons, Doctors, and Disease

psychiatrist carefully notes that there is no evidence that cannabis causes severe organic disease like alcohol. It also produces less impairment of driving than alcohol. The most serious charge leveled against the drug is that it may induce personality or psychotic disorders. Psychiatrists in Morocco, India, Egypt, Nigeria say that marihuana may incite insanity. Benabud of Morocco declares it causes a condition for which he has coined the name "cannabis psychosis."

There is just as much violent controversy among psychiatrists over marihuana as there is among other physicians and the public in general. Some psychiatrists disagree with Benabud about the precipitation of psychoses by marihuana. Bromberg, an American psychiatrist, believes that the cause of some of his psychotic patients' illnesses is marihuana toxicity. It could also be true that the cannabis precipitated a latent condition. The subject is highly controversial and probably won't be settled for a long time. Years ago psychiatrists Allentuck and Bowman concluded from their studies that marihuana will not induce psychosis in a well adjusted stable person. One could also use the same argument for alcoholics. We could also ask why would a well adjusted stable person use drugs?

Grinspoon raised the very intriguing question as to whether or not *marihuana might protect* some people *against psychoses*. His argument is that more neurotics and personality disordered individuals use the drug than does the general population. If so, then we should expect more psychoses in these people. But the incidence, he says, is not higher, which might indicate that mentally disturbed persons may get some protection from the use of cannabis. This possibility, of course, needs proof. To advocate marihuana, at this time, to prevent possible nervous breakdowns would be treated as heresy and excommunication from one's community.

Interestingly, very early in this century, cannabis was used to get drug addicts off narcotics, alcohol, barbituates, and chloral hydrate. Then the patients were taken off cannabis because it is not addictive. This therapy was utilized by Allentuck and Bowman in 1942 and again by Thompson and Proctor in 1953. Should it be tried again?

In a poor country like India there are no legal restrictions to using marihuana. Large numbers of people employ cannabis to escape from hardship and poverty—to escape reality and pursue the high.

Drugs, Demons, Doctors, and Disease

In the USA, for many years, the ghettos were the main consumers of marihuana. Today the use is very widespread and is the in-thing for many students. A great number have tried cannabis purely for curiosity, because their friends are using it, and they want to see what this high trip is all about. For some it is an attempt to find themselves, to explore in depth who and what they are, to "expand their minds," even to find God.

Others are revolting against society, and, because cannabis is illegal, are using it to flaunt society. "Turning on" is rapidly increasing in the armed forces, and the army high command states that black troops have a larger percentage of marihuana users than do white troops. The drug for many is an escape from feelings of personal frustrations, inadequacy, anxiety and depression.

New York college drug users described themselves as anxious, moody, cynical, disgusted, impulsive, rebellious, and restless—significantly more so than nonusers. They also admit never being ambitious or secure. Seventeen percent took illegal drugs including LSD, and used amphetamines more than any other group. Tranquilizers were taken also. Most had limited or no experience with heroin, opiates, or cocaine. Twenty six percent of the students used amphetamines, barbiturates, or tranquilizers, but no illegal drugs. They were greater consumers of tranquilizers than the illicit drug users and the majority had physicians' prescriptions for their drugs.

David Popoff records a survey in 1970 of 14,748 respondents to a questionnaire on drugs in *Psychology Today*. Forty seven percent tried marihuana, 18 percent LSD, 98 percent coffee, tea and aspirin, 46 percent use tobacco and 14 percent drink alcohol every day. Ten percent use sedatives and amphetamines at least once a week, while 11 percent have tried heroin or cocaine at least once.

Sixty percent of regular marihuana devotees also are tobacco smokers. However, only 26 percent of daily tobacco smokers use marihuana once a week, while 42 percent have never tried it. Heavy marihuana users also take LSD, amphetamines and opiates more often than light users.

There is a very close relationship between marihuana and LSD. Interesting figures are available. Only 1 percent of non-marihuana users have ever taken LSD; however, 31 percent of once-a-month marihuana users, 58 percent of once-a-week marihuana users, and

77 percent of daily marihuana users have tried LSD and other hallucinogenic agents.

Fourteen percent of daily marihuana users have taken opiates more than once or twice. Infrequent users of marihuana seldom try opiates.

Clark and Funkhouser, in a similar survey of physicians and researchers on psychedelic drugs, found that professional researchers consider them less dangerous and more therapeutically promising than do non-researchers. They do not regard them as "unmitigated blessings." In fact, the researchers do not agree among themselves as to the dangers of the drugs and the legal status of marihuana. They do believe, however, that there has been an exaggeration of the dangers of LSD.

OPIATES

Opium comes from the plant called Papaver somniferum, the sleep producing poppy. The best opium comes from Turkey, and is derived from the dried milky juice of the unripe pod of the plant. The important alkaloid chemicals of opium are morphine and heroin.

Opium has been used for thousands of years. DeQuincey called it the panacea for all human woes and the secret of happiness. While temporarily it may fulfill such promises, in chronic users it brings all the dire miseries accruing to addicts. While morphine is difficult to get, except by prescription, heroin is sold illegally and the cost is usually so high, that addicts must resort to crime to support their habit. Like marihuana, it is frequently adulterated by unscrupulous pushers, thereby causing toxicity and sometimes death. Marihuana is sometimes "spiked" with heroin to "hook" the user to the hard narcotic.

Psychiatrist John Ball of Philadelphia indicates that there were more than 108,000 *known* opiate addicts in January 1970 with 77% of them in the New York, California, Illinois area. Other estimates have placed as many as 100,000 heroin addicts in New York City alone. Heroin is the principal drug of abuse with morphine, Dilaudid®, paregoric, codeine, Demerol® (meperidine), and Dolophine® (methadone), following in this order. Ball claims that opiate addiction is highest in blacks, Mexicans, and Puerto Ricans in the USA general population. In addition to the major groups of addicters, there are minor groups such as musicians, doctors, nurses, artists, prostitutes, and pushers.

We will only consider heroin here, as it is the main opiate used. It may be taken by sniffing or intravenous injection. It is a powerful pain killer and a good general sedative. Strangely, morphine was introduced to combat opium addiction without realizing it was an addicting drug itself. Later, heroin was introduced to fight morphine and opium addiction and it too proved to be another habit forming medication.

Heroin, when taken into the body, produces an easing of worries, fears, and tension. A high follows, along with inactivity, causing a stuporous like mood. Pupils are constricted. There is a diminution of appetite, thirst and sex drive. Pain is reduced or lost, so that the individual may be unaware of pain caused by appendicitis, pleurisy, or other serious disease. The pulse and respiratory rate are slowed. The persistent user is hooked on the drug and is called a "junkie."

Certain serious complications may accompany heroin usage. Phlebitis or clotted veins follows repeated injections. Cases of spinal cord destruction with paralysis and death have been reported. Hepatitis or liver disease may result from using a contaminated unsterilized needle of another junkie. Malaria, syphilis, and many infectious diseases have been transmitted by similar means. Pushers cut heroin often with cheaper drugs and talc. When these mixtures are injected, severe and lethal reactions may take place. Death frequently follows an overdose with a heroin content stronger than the individual has been accustomed to taking. Usually, a tolerance to the drug calls for larger doses to get the high, and so the habit becomes more expensive to support.

An addict failing to get his "fix" will soon get withdrawal symptoms. This state is accompanied by chills, nervousness, insomnia, vomiting, diarrhea, aches, pains, tremors and sometimes convulsions. Unless heroin is given, the patient will continue to go through this "cold turkey" condition until exhausted. However, medical treatment makes the withdrawal more comfortable.

Treatment advocated today, for those earnestly desiring to get off heroin or other opiates, is the methadone method. This drug satisfies the craving for opiates and can be given orally, thereby replacing the hard narcotic. Later an attempt can be made to get the patient off methadone. Withdrawal symptoms are much milder with methadone than heroin. The drug is given at a clinic, for supervisory reasons, and the patient returns to a gainful occupation. The cost of the medication is cheap and therefore the need to steal for maintaining an expensive heroin addicition, is gone. Because the patient must return to the clinic to get his medication, psychologic observation of the addict is possible and social rehabilitation is more probable. A. D. Stutchin of Paterson, New Jersey, has treated over 5,000 addicts with methadone and attained excellent results. However, they were people who sought help for their habit, and efforts to reclaim individuals of this type is more successful.

Another treatment available is that of utilizing narcotic antagonists, such as naloxone or cyclazocine, which diminish or prevent entirely the narcotic effects of dependency or overdosage. Unlike methadone therapy, it does not substitute one habituating drug for another. Psychiatrist Max Fink of New York City believes that naloxone is the superior medication and advocates implanting the drug under the skin for slow longtime release to block heroin dependency for months.

A third method of treatment is that of group therapy, which is given at centers devoted to handling the drug problem. Places that have received recognition are Synanon, Daytop, Corona Rehabilitation Center, and the New York City Addiction Services Agency.

THE HALLUCINOGENS

LSD ("acid") and other drugs such as peyote and mescaline ("cactus") and psilocybine ("magic mushroom") are not physically addictive and usually not physically harmful. The danger is that nobody knows when he is going to react adversely under their influence. The fact that one has had "good trips" is no guarantee that the next one might not cause him to jump out a window. Psychiatrist Daniel Freedman of Chicago describes the hallucinogens as causing the user to focus overwhelmingly on his subjective sensations and their meaning to him, while neglecting the importance of everyday reality.

LSD (lysergic acid diethylamide) may produce terrifying trips with marked psychotic paranoid symptoms. These episodes may last for many hours. A single bad trip may recur in flashbacks weeks, months, or years later.

Strange effects are noted when LSD is given to animals. Cats become afraid of mice. Spiders weave abnormal webs. Rats and mice develop fever, while pigeons have subnormal temperatures. Pigeons become withdrawn and catatonic, while dogs turn aggressive. Siamese fighting fish swim backards, and the skin of guppy fish becomes darkened.

LSD penetrates the brain cells and, as it does, the amount of serotonin increases in the cells. While this is happening, behavior begins to change. An electroencephalogram or brain wave recording shows activity in the midbrain. Just how LSD causes its unusual effects is not clear. Donald Luria of Cornell University Medical College believes that there is no place for the experimental use of LSD in medicine or psychiatry, but there is need for further study of the drug in three areas where it has shown some promise of good, namely, alcoholism, psychoneurosis, and terminal disease such as cancer.

The hallucinogen-tripper experiences beautiful fantastic colors which he never visualized before. Senses become so acute that he can now taste sound and hear light. The environment merges with the individual and he feels that he and the objects are one and the same. This brings him close to the universe and God. Time, space and the body become twisted and distorted while the sense of individuality disappears. Apparitions of famous religious personages appear. There is also a marked erotic overlay to the hallucinations. Appearing, too, are unpleasant sights such as hideous-shaped animals, snakes, octopuses, maggots and horrible crawling things.

Many important claims are made for the usage of LSD by its worshipers. Creativity, aesthetic sensitivity, and insight into one's personality are supposed to be improved by taking acid. There is no evidence that this ever really happens. It has also been said that the capacity to give or receive love is intensified by LSD. However, the acid experience is self centered and intensely personal, the antithesis of the love concept, a pure illusion. Equally unfounded is the claim that the drug is an aphrodisiac. It might cause mental erotic hallucinations, but there is no physical backup. Hence it is actually an anti-aphrodisiac.

The possibility has been expressed that LSD may enable the

user to communicate with Christ, religious figures, or even God. (The Indians took hallucinogens before conversing with their gods.) Yet there is no evidence in the lives of the indulgers of LSD, that there has been a real religious transcendence or that their lives have been altered in any way.

There is no denying the fact that for many people the high stimulated by acid is pleasant. Nevertheless, the ensuing cost for some may not be worth the pleasure. They suffer overwhelming panic, hideous illusions, the horrible fear of insanity, suicides, homicides, possible chromosome damage, temporary or permanent psychoses. The long range effects of LSD are still to be determined. In the last few years we have finally learned what the long range results of smoking are. It would be too much to expect that one can abuse the delicate brain repeatedly with powerful chemicals and not find eventually some disorganization or disintegration.

COCAINE—AMPHETAMINES AND BARBITURATES

Cocaine existed before amphetamines. It still is, and probably will continue to be used by those consecrated to stimulation. The drug is derived from the coca bush of South America. Its medical employment has already been discussed. Cocaine is either sniffed up into the nose or injected. It gives the user a feeling of pleasure and exhilaration. When it wears off the addict may feel great fear and alarm. South American Indians use it for increasing their endurance while working. Addicts sometimes combine it with heroin to get up and down jolts. This is known as "Speedball."

More commonly taken in this country are the synthetic amphetamines, such as Benzedrine®, Dexedrine®, Desoxyn®, and Methedrine®. They are legally prescribed by physicians to curb appetites and sleepiness, to increase energy, relieve minor depression, and treat narcolepsy, a disease in which the patients find it difficult to stay awake. Amphetamines, known also as "ups" and "speed," produce increased alertness. For this reason, they are used by truck drivers to keep awake while on the road and by students who stay up nights to study for examinations.

Heavy oral use or injection of speed causes overconfidence, aggressiveness, hallucinations, and psychotic episodes. Continued abuse may result in aggressive behavior, loss of appetite, tremors, shakiness, headaches, silly behavior, and paleness. Research findings indicate that amphetamines increase noradrenalin at nerve cell junctions. This is noted in brain regions associated with heart action, moods, and vigilance. The dangers from continued injections of ups are inability to sleep, high blood pressure, rapid heart rate and irregular heart beats, suspicious and violent behavior. With the "speed freak" there is deterioration of all values, and he will do anything to get his drugs. "Speed" causes death in overdosed individuals.

Barbiturates are legitimately prescribed for sedation, high blood pressure, epilepsy, and insomnia. Abuse or heavy use, either orally or by injection, gives rise to depression, dullness, confusion, drunken appearance and staggering gait, blurring of speech and death. Barbiturates are called "downs," and also by the color of the various capsules. Abrupt withdrawal from an addict may cause death. There are individuals who alternate between ups and downs, and who take heroin too. Barbiturates and alcohol may be a very deadly combination.

The search for kicks has wandered far afield from the drugs described here. It has involved sniffing and inhalation of glue, lacquer, gasoline, Freon®, paint thinner, lighter and cleaning fluids, solvents, aerosols, insecticides, nose drops and in fact whatever can be inhaled for a supposed high. Ingested material may include anything, even such bizarre items as aspirin and Coca Cola®, beer and antivertigo tablets, cold medicines, nutmeg, cough medicines, heart stimulants and asthma remedies, and throat disks.

A considerable number of drug users are getting fed up with the psychedelic life. As dissatisfaction spreads they have abandoned drugs and gone over to religion. They are now turned on to Christ and are zealously evangelizing their confreres. Known as Jesus freaks, they are experiencing a new high, one which gives joy and happiness without the complications that drug abuse brings.

Is the drug scene a passing fancy, or a permanent passion? For many, undoubtedly, it is a temporary indulgence, a curiosity, a desire to be one of the crowd. For others whose desire is to escape reality, the craze for drugs becomes the only way of life. Does anyone benefit from the drug scene? Yes! the manufacturers, wholesalers, legal and illegal dealers do. Does the user, abuser, or addict benefit? The nonindulger, the law, and the medical profession definitely say no! Therefore, their prime purpose is to educate and prevent new youngsters and adults from participating

Drugs, Demons, Doctors, and Disease

in this habit. Their second important interest is to get off drugs individuals who can be salvaged. It must be emphatically stressed that one can get high and find happiness through other media. Perhaps this argument may finally prevail, if we are really rational creatures. For the brain is a complex organ, and the drugs scrambling its units and circuits may do irreparable damage.

For the devotees of expanding the mind, there is now on the horizon something new without drugs. For years Zen and yogi meditators have altered body functions by sheer force of will. Wired to electroencephalogram machines now, there is evidence they can change the pattern of their own brain waves. Individuals, too, can see their own brain waves on various types of recently developed screens. By mental manipulation, it is claimed the subjects can be taught to change their own wave patterns for the betterment of themselves, thus altering or expanding their minds. The ramifications are tremendous if this proves to be factual and develops under scientific control and research.

Chapter Eleven

RESPIRATORY TRACT, EYE AND CARDIOVASCULAR DRUGS

THE RESPIRATORY TRACT or breathing system begins with the nose and ends in the alveoli or smallest lung units. The purpose of this system is to bring air into the lungs from which oxygen can be extracted, and to discharge carbon dioxide from the lungs into the exhaled air. Anything that interferes with this function may cause temporary or permanent damage or even death.

As the air is contaminated with many pollutants today, persons breathing it are being constantly exposed to more respiratory disorders. The subject of pollution and allergy will be discussed later, but for now we will consider the most common maladies to which this system is subjected.

HEAD COLDS

Head colds (acute rhinitis) and acute sinusitis are usually provoked by viruses or bacteria. Treatment is either directed towards relieving the symptoms or to attacking the microorganisms responsible for the illness. For relief of symptoms, most prescriptions contain drugs like aspirin and phenacetin. Sometimes caffeine is added to the preparations to give an uplift to the depressing discomfort. Antihistamines may be given alone, or combined with the above medications. Such a combination is Coricidin®.

Nasal decongestants, to shrink down swollen membranes, are

given as nose drops, tablets or capsules. Among such preparations are ephedrine, Propadrine®, Dimetapp®, Naldecon®, Biomydrin®, Otrivin®, Tyzine®, Benzedrex®, Neo-Synephrine®, and Afrin®. Virus colds do not respond to antibiotics, but bacterial colds may. Secondary bacterial infections frequently accompany viral infections, and will usually respond to proper medication.

Sore throats caused by acute pharyngitis or tonsillitis are produced by a number of organisms, but the streptococcus is one of the most common incitants. To relieve the sore throat, hot gargles are prescribed along with analgesics to reduce pain and fever. Anesthetic-antibiotic throat lozenges are sometimes helpful. Antibiotics or sulfa drugs are effective in halting the infection. Laryngitis is often treated with steam inhalations in addition to the above therapy.

Middle ear infections frequently follow colds, especially in young children. There is usually pain and a fullness in the involved ear. If treated early, it may not be necessary to open the ear drum to drain pus. Anti-infective agents will ordinarily control the infection. Ear drops may be instilled to relieve congestion and pain in the inflamed ear drum. Such medications are Auralgan®, Otic Domeboro® solution, Neo-Cortef Ear Drops®, Neodecadron Solution®, and Biomydrin Otic®. The external ear is also subjected to direct infection by bacteria and fungi. Treatment is accordingly.

EYE DISORDERS

Because the eyes are anatomically closely associated with the nose and sinuses, infections may directly invade the eyes from this region. Another common affliction is conjunctivitis (inflammation of external membrane of the eye). However, this ailment can also occur from direct contact with infection from an external source. Anti-infective agents such as NeoDecadron®, Neo-Cortef®, Neo-Medrol®, or other medications can be applied to the eyes. Ulcers occasionally develop in the eyes because of infection and they will respond to antimicrobial medications. Glaucoma, a frequent eye malady, is not due to infection, but rather to abnormal pressure buildup in the eyes. If treatment is delayed, partial or permanent loss of sight may occur. Drugs which relieve this pressure are pilocarpine, phystigmine, and the synthetics carbachol and demecarium.

ACUTE BRONCHITIS

A cold which migrates down into the bronchial tubes from the throat is known as acute bronchitis. This may clear up by itself or with medication. If not, the condition may become chronic with resulting permanent damage. In acute bronchitis there may be a dry irritative cough, following which a scanty thick sputum or phlegm may be raised. The sputum gradually becomes more abundant and yellowish.

Antibiotics are usually effectual in terminating acute bacterial bronchitis. Expectorants may also be employed to loosen thick sputum or phlegm so that it may be coughed up more easily. Potassium iodide and ammonium chloride have been prescribed for this purpose for many years. Inhalations of Alevaire® and Mucomyst® are of value because they have a detergent action on the bronchial mucous membranes. When wheezing is present and severe, an anti-asthmatic drug is ordered. Coughing, if constant, may irritate the bronchial tubes and cause marked discomfort. Some of the drugs which can be administered to relieve it are Tessalon®, Nectadon®, Romilar®, Dimetane Expectorant®, Triaminic Expectorant®, and Benylin Expectorant®. Older remedies are elixir of terpin hydrate, Stoke's expectorant, and brown mixture.

BRONCHIECTASIS

Bronchiectasis is a disease in which there is dilation, outpocketings, and degeneration of the bronchial tubes. This condition may follow bronchopneumonia, foreign bodies lodged in the tubes and causing obstruction, compression of the tubes by cancer or enlarged glands, tuberculosis, lung abscess, or bronchial cancer. Cough is the predominant symptom. Repeated attacks of pneumonia may occur in this area, and the patient may occasionally cough up some blood. The quantity of sputum the patient raises may be enormous. It is usually greenish or yellowish in color. Diagnosis is made on history, x-ray, and bronchoscopic examination of the tubes with an electrically lighted instrument called a bronchoscope. The most common type of bronchietasis follows bronchitis, bronchopneumonia, foreign body and tuberculosis. Our discussion of treatment will be for this kind of bronchietasis.

Surgical removal of diseased lung tissue, if it is well localized, may result in cure. Otherwise, treatment is medical and includes expectorants and antibiotics. Certain positions, used by the patient morning and night and known as postural drainage, enable him to bring up large quantities of sputum from the diseased bronchial tubes. When successful, this procedure gives him freedom from continual coughing during the day. To facilitate this clearance, bronchial dilating agents such as Isuprel® or Vaponefren®, and decongesting drugs like Neo-Synephrine®, are administered by nebulizers before starting postural drainage. Some physicians also employ detergent and mucolytic (mucus splitting) drugs. Orally given bronchodilators containing ephedrine are valuable too. Antibiotics help to keep infection under control.

CHRONIC BRONCHITIS AND EMPHYSEMA

Chronic bronchitis is a very common disease. Many people have only mild symptoms such as a morning cough, with some raising of sputum, and do not seek medical care. Eventually, when and if the disorder becomes severe, and the condition not reversible, then they ardently seek help. There is a very definite association between cigarette smoking and chronic bronchitis. Frequently, the elimination of smoking clears the cough and bronchitis. However, not all cases of chronic bronchitis are caused by smoking. Certain occupations, where the workers inhale dusts, chemical fumes, and other irritants, may produce this disorder. Asthma and cystic fibrosis are additional factors in producing chronic bronchitis.

Treatment consists, initially, of eliminating any incitants which may have given rise to the condition such as smoking, occupational hazards, or allergens. For relief, bronchodilators, decongestants, expectorants and antibiotics are prescribed. The bronchodilator ephedrine is frequently combined with the expectorant iodide in preparations such as Tedral® and Quadrinal®. Amesec® and Marax® contain ephedrine but no iodide.

Emphysema often occurs along with chronic bronchitis. The principal finding in emphysema is destruction of the alveoli or terminal units of the lung. No treatment can replace this lost lung tissue. Eventually, if the disease continues to progress, there is insufficient lung tissue available to support life. Most patients with emphysema are heavy cigarette smokers, and also live in heavily-polluted air environments.

The treatment of emphysema is similar to chronic bronchitis for the two are closely associated. Antibiotics are needed in addition to the oral bronchodilators mentioned above. Nebulized bronchodilators may also have to be employed such as Medihaler®, Isuprel Mistometer®, Duo-Medihaler®, and Metermatic Vaponefrin®. Theophylline is an excellent drug for use to relieve difficult breathing and wheezing. It can be given orally as Choledyl® or Elixophyllin®, by rectal enema as Fleet's theophylline rectal unit, as aminophylline rectal suppositories, or intravenously. The oral expectorants used in chronic bronchitis are valuable in emphysema, too. Postural drainage may have to be instituted. In the final stages of the disease, oxygen may have to be administered to prolong life.

PNEUMONIA

There is no specific treatment for viral pneumonias. If one accepts the mycoplasma as large viruses (rather than small bacteria) then these microbes respond to antibiotics. What we will consider now are the bacterial pneumonias. In pneumonia there may or may not be chest pain. The symptoms are similar to those of acute bronchitis—for actually pneumonia is an extension of bronchitis into the lungs. The patient usually has a cough, shortness of breath, expectoration of sputum, fever, rapid pulse, and possibly hypoxia (lack of oxygen), because there is less lung tissue available to absorb oxygen and the demands of the body tissues increase.

There are certain bacteria which cause most of the pneumonias, namely, the pneumococci, streptococci, hemophilus influenzae, Klebsiella pneumoniae and gram negative bacilli. Antibiotics are used which will be effective against the microorganisms, after prior sensitivity testing. Expectorants, cough suppressors, bronchodilators, oxygen, antipyretics (fever lowering drugs), may or may not be used, depending upon the judgement of the physician. Complications, if they arise, such as lung abscess, pleurisy, and empyema (pus in the chest) are treated accordingly.

PULMONARY EDEMA

Pulmonary edema is a swelling of the lungs due to fluid leaking into the lungs from the blood circulating in the organ. It may be produced by heart failure, pneumonia, or lung destruction (infarct). The victim complains of shortness of breath, pain in the chest, cough, bloody and frothy sputum. He can easily go into shock and die. Mild attacks disappear by themselves, but severe ones may kill. If the patient is suffering from heart failure, morphine or Demerol® may be given. Oxygen is helpful, if given under pressure, to help force the fluid back into the blood stream. Tourniquets may be applied to the extremities, in rotary fashion, to reduce the amount of blood coming to the heart, thereby decreasing its work load.

If pneumonia is the cause of the edema, sedatives may be used, but the cough reflex must not be abolished. Otherwise the patient will be unable to raise the fluids and will drown in his own frothy sputum. Oxygen will be given if needed. Antibiotics must be vigorously utilized, as they are the sheet anchor for clearing the pneumonia organisms.

PULMONARY INFARCTS

Pulmonary infarcts are very common and are due to the death of lung tissue caused by an obstructed artery, whose circulation has been cut off by a blood clot traveling to the lung (pulmonary embolism) from the heart or from a leg vein. If the clots are very tiny there may be no symptoms. If large, there may be severe reactions and even instant death. The usual symptoms of lung infarcts are pain in the chest, cough, the raising of blood tinged sputum, and possibly shock.

For immediate therapy morphine or Demerol® is given to ease the pain. Oxygen is administered to treat hypoxia (lack of oxygen). Atropine® may be given by injection to stop bronchial spasms and the oozing of fluids into the lung (pulmonary edema).

To prevent clots from further damaging the lung and possibly killing the patient, anticoagulant medication may be started, using heparin by injection and then following up with the slower acting coumarin. If the source of the clot is located in the lower extremities, the surgeon can tie off the veins involved. Surgical attempts are made, in life saving emergencies, to remove a large clot from the lung by special gadgets introduced into the circulation and guided into the lungs under x-ray fluoroscopic control. The clot is grasped, removed, and the obstruction immediately relieved. A new method to digest lung clots by injection of urokinase and streptokinase enzymes into the blood stream, is being tried.

According to a report in 1971 by Shafer and Duboff of New York, blood clots traveling to the lungs kill 4 to 10% of individuals dying in general hospitals, 20 to 25% dying in chronic disease hospitals, and 30 to 50% of patients who die of heart disease. Pulmonary embolisms are the most common acute lung disorders in the general adult population. The chief cause of post-operative deaths and chest complications is post-operative pulmonary embolisms.

THE HEART

The heart is a four-chambered pump designed for propelling blood throughout the body in an enclosed system of blood vessels. The rate of beating is determined by a coordinated conducting system in the heart which is influenced by two sets of nerves, one which accelerates and the other decelerates the conducting system.

Sometimes there are abnormal rhythms and irregular beating of the heart. They may be of minor consequence or they may have a serious implication. The physician determines the course of action. Drugs administered for correcting these disorders are digitalis, propranolol hydrochloride, quinidine, Pronestyl® (procainamide), and Xylocaine® (lidocaine).

CONGESTIVE HEART FAILURE

Congestive heart failure, also a very common condition, indicates that the biological pump is failing. The two lower and most important chambers of the heart are the ventricles. When they are unable to pump out their full complement of blood, there is a backing-up of the circulation. This affects the entire body. A well known symptom is swelling of the feet and legs. The lungs are also congested and the patient has symptoms of shortness of breath (dyspnea), cyanosis or oxygen lack, cough, nervousness, and loss of appetite. The patient cannot lie flat in bed but must be propped up with pillows.

There are a number of reasons for congestive heart failure such as thyroid disease, beriberi (lack of vitamin B_1), congenital heart defects, high blood pressure (hypertension), heart disease, including coronary artery disease, anemia, lung diseases and other maladies.

Treatment should be directed towards combating the inciting factors. Thyroid disease and beriberi can be successfully treated.

Congenital (birth-defect) heart disease may be surgically remedied. Anemia reduces the amount of oxygen reaching the heart and, if corrected, the heart will recover. Coronary artery disease decreases blood flow to the heart muscle. Treatment is either medical or surgical to relieve the obstruction.

For heart failure itself, certain measures are instituted to improve the pumping ability of the heart muscle. The main drug given is digitalis, which was discovered in the 18th century by Withering. Strophanthus, discovered by Frazer in 1890, is prescribed for patients who cannot tolerate digitalis. Squills, known to the ancient Egyptians, is seldom used anymore. Formerly the powedered leaf and the tincture (alcoholic extract) of digitalis were administered. Newer preparations are digoxin, digitoxin, and lanatoside (Cedilanid C®). Oubain, derived from strophanthus, is occasionally utilized for its rapid action. The type of drug and the method of prescribing is determined by the physician. Side effects encountered with digitalis are nausea, vomiting, headache, drowsiness, slow pulse, visual disturbances and delirium.

Digitalis strengthens the heart muscle and its improved functioning usually reduces tissue swelling. Diuretics however are utilized along with digitalis to remove salt and water. One of these drugs is mercury, which was known to Paracelsus in the 10th century in the form of calomel and which is also a laxative. The organic mercurials have replaced this preparation and they act more effectively in an acid urine. So ammonium chloride may be given to acidify the urine. Aminophylline, intravenously, also intensifies mercurial diuresis. Mercurials are best administered by injection. Among these compounds are Mercuhydrin® (meralluride), Mercupurin® (mercurophylline) and Thiomerin® (mercaptomerin). Side effects or mercury poisoning produce stomatitis (inflamed mouth), nausea, vomiting, diarrhea, abdominal pain, blood in the urine, kidney damage, shock and possibly death.

Also used for kidney diuresis are the thiazide drugs—Diuril®, Hydrodiuril®, Esidrex®, Enduron®, and Renese®. When administered, one must be on guard that too much potassium is not lost from the body. Otherwise, symptoms of potassium depletion will appear such as nausea, vomiting, lethargy, muscle cramps and lowered blood pressure. The intake of potassium-containing foods must be increased to equalize the loss.

More powerful diuretics are available, if needed, like Edecrin®

and Lasix®. Aldactone® has a different diuretic action. It inhibits the action of the hormone aldosterone, thereby preventing the kidneys from reabsorbing sodium. This mineral is responsible for retaining excessive water in the tissues. Sodium is present in common salt which is sodium chloride. Salt must be restricted in congestive heart failure.

The treatment of congestive heart failure is similar to that of pulmonary edema and includes sedation with morphine or Demerol®, the giving of oxygen, using rotating tourniquets to reduce blood flow to the heart, phlebotomy or bleeding of the patient to decrease blood volume, water and salt restriction to stop tissue and organ engorgement. If fluid collects in the chest, it can be removed by a number of methods. If drugs fail to stop cardiac arrhythmias, electric shock known as cardioversion, may be applied to the heart. For irregular beats and rhythms are an added burden to a faltering heart.

ANGINA PECTORIS

Another very common heart disorder is angina pectoris, usually described as pain in the chest, and associated, in the layman's mind, with heart pain. Actually, the word more specifically means a strangling in the chest. The patients suffering from this affliction state that they experience a choking (with or without pain), a severe tightness or a hard compression or a smothering sensation in the chest, and finally a fear of impending death. Anginal pain may radiate to the left arm and down to the fingers, or it may go up into the left side of neck, both sides of the neck, and even to the right arm or abdomen. Basically, angina is a cry of agony from the heart pleading for more oxygen.

There are a number of reasons for angina pectoris. The most common is disease of the coronary arteries, which supply the heart with blood. Coronary artery disease (conorary atherosclerosis) is due mainly to fatty deposits in the arterial walls. The portion of the heart muscle supplied by the artery cries out for oxygen, when the demand on the muscle exceeds the diminishing trickle of blood being given to it. As the process continues to advance, the blood vessel finally becomes occluded. Coronary disease may be diagnosed by history, physical examination, electrocardiographic studies, and x-ray visualization of the coronary arteries by special injection techniques.

Drugs, Demons, Doctors, and Disease

In some cases of angina, however, there is no evidence of coronary arterial disease. According to cardiologist Richard Gorlin of Boston, 10 to probably 20% of angina individuals will show no atherosclerosis, even though they have angina and have had cardiac infarction (heart muscle death). The cause is not quite clear. One suggestion is that a clot forms long enough to occlude the artery and then quickly dissolves and disappears. In cases of anemia, thyroid disease and other types of heart disease, angina may also occur in the presence of normal coronary arteries. If the underlying malady can be corrected, the symptoms of angina may be relieved. Atherosclerosis is the main cause of the disease and the leading cause of disability and death in the USA.

Certain risk factors are associated with the cause and aggravation of coronary disease. They are smoking, diabetes, hypertension (high blood pressure), and disorders of lipid (fat) metabolism. If smoking is stopped completely, the risk of sudden death is drastically diminished and relief from angina is dramatic. Reduction of high blood pressure will alleviate angina. Correction of certain lipid (fat) disorders, especially those known as Type II and Type IV, is helpful in relieving coronary atherosclerotic disease.

Type II is characterized by high blood cholesterol and is treated with a low cholesterol diet, reduction in saturated fats (hard fats), and an increase in consumption of polyunsaturated fats (oils). Drugs used to lower cholesterol are clofibrate, d-thyroxine, cholestyramine, nicotinic acid, and estrogens. Type IV shows a mild increase in cholesterol and a marked increase in triglycerides (a chemical combination of glycerol with three fatty acids). The glucose (sugar) tolerance test (for detecting diabetes) is abnormal which indicates that Type IV lipid (fat) disorder is due to some carbohydrate abnormality. Restriction of carbohydrates in the diet, mainly sugar, helps to improve the situation. Clofibrate and weight reduction is of value too.

Angina can be relieved by reducing activity to one's heart capacity. The prime remedy used to treat the discomfort is nitroglycerine. Tablets are placed under the tongue to be absorbed from there. To treat and prevent attacks, the patient always carries the drug with him. He may take the nitroglycerine before exertion such as climbing stairs, walking a distance, sexual activity and any other physical stress or strain. Emotional upsets and exposure to cold also precipitate angina. Sedatives or tranquilizers may be advised for emotion-packed situations, although avoidance is preferable. Amyl nitrate along with nitroglycerine have been the principal drugs given for angina for more than 100 years. Newer drugs are Propranolol®, Isordril®, and Peritrate®. In severe angina, not responding to these agents, morphine or Demerol® may be used. Some people have benefited from large doses of Vitamin E, others claim it has no value.

MYOCARDIAL INFARCTION

The end result of angina pectoris, produced by disease of the coronary arteries, is death of the heart muscle (myocardial infarction) being supplied by the particular coronary artery. This sudden shutdown is the common heart attack and it claims many victims each year in our country.

With final occlusion of the artery, the heart muscle (myocardium) cries out with severe angina for oxygen but the cry is in vain. There is no response to nitroglycerine. The muscle begins to die. The patient may go into shock, with symptoms described previously under this subject. Depending upon the severity of the attack, the patient dies quickly, or, if he does not, the final issue may be in doubt for quite a while as to whether he will die or recover. The great majority of persons survive the initial heart attack but succumb eventually to another attack. The difference, many times, between living and dying is the speed with which the patient gets medical attention.

The best place for the heart patient is in the coronary care unit of a hospital. Emergency care at home or in the ambulance is directed towards relieving angina with morphine or Demerol®. Atropine® is used to prevent arrhythmias and slow the heart rate, lidocaine (Xylocaine®) to stop irregular beats when they appear, oxygen to relieve hypoxia (lack of oxygen).

When the patient gets into the coronary care unit, all vital signs are carefully monitored. In case of heart stoppage, adrenalin or calcium gluconate is injected into the heart to restore beating. Irregular beats may cause heart stoppage and death. The physician may use Lidocaine®, propranolol, and other drugs for this emergency. Oxygen is often effective in relieving dyspnea, and slowing the fast heart rate. Whether other drugs such as digitalis, quinidine, and anticoagulants should be employed depends upon the physician's judgement.

RHEUMATIC HEART DISEASE

One of the most frightening childhood diseases, before the advent of antibiotics, was rheumatic fever and rheumatic heart disease. Crippling of the heart was and is the most dreaded complication of rheumatic fever. However, even adults may develop this rheumatic affliction.

The disease follows a streptococcus infection of the throat, sinuses, tonsils or other areas. The reactions to this organism are believed to be allergic in nature. The disease is characterized by fever, migrating arthritis and rashes. Heart involvement may be obvious or subtle, with damage to the muscle, valves, or outer lining of the heart (pericardium). If severe, the patient may go into heart failure and die.

Treatment of rheumatic fever has consisted chiefly of the use of salicylates to reduce fever and relieve the pain of arthritis. Such drugs are aspirin, aspirin compounds, sodium salicylate, and salicylamide. The drugs do not halt the disease. Penicillin, which acts to eliminate the streptococcus, is given in large doses. Some patients are put on penicillin continuously, to avoid future attacks of rheumatic fever and further heart damage. If the person is allergic to penicillin, erythromycin is substituted. The corticosteroids (cortisone derivatives) may be used to temporarily block the destructive action of the disease on the heart.

HYPERTENSION

Hypertension or high blood pressure is defined as an elevation of either the upper blood pressure, which occurs with each heart beat and is called the systolic blood pressure, or the lower and constant pressure, which exists between beats, and is called the diastolic blood pressure. Usually 90mm of mercury is accepted as the upper limit for the diastolic pressure and 140mm of mercury for the systolic pressure. However, these figures are only relative, for age and other factors must be taken into consideration when blood pressure readings are taken. Hypertension decreases life expectancy. Lowering high blood pressure increases life expectancy.

Blood pressure rises for many reasons. Hypertension may only be temporary as for example when a patient goes to see his doctor and gets uptight. Blood pressure rises, too, when a person becomes frightened, anxious, angry, and aggressive. This elevation again is only temporary. What we are mainly concerned with is hypertensive disease.

Organic causes for hypertension are chiefly kidney and adrenal disorders, toxic thyroid disease, overactive pituitary and parathyroid glands, toxemia of pregnancy, hemorrhages of the brain and stricture of the aorta, which is the artery leading out of the left side of the heart. Females taking contraceptive pills often develop hypertension which subsides when the pills are stopped.

Surgery on the adrenal glands and kidneys often causes high blood pressure to return to normal. The same is true for surgical operations on the thyroid and parathyroid glands and also the aorta. Toxemia of pregnancy responds to medical treatment or to terminating the pregnancy.

Where surgery is not indicated, various drugs are used to bring down blood pressure. The rauwolfias, sedatives and tranquilizers are given for mild hypertension. In these cases reduction of anxiety and nervous tension is usually enough to get the pressure back to normal. In more resistant cases other drugs are administered. Nitroprusside®, Diazoxide® and hydralazine dilate blood vessels and thus lower hypertension. Methyl dopa accomplishes the same purpose by blocking certain chemicals in tissues, like noradrenalin, which elevate blood pressure. Guanethidine is also antagonistic to noradrenalin. Hexamethonium blocks stimulating nerve impulses across nerve ganglia, causing blood pressure to drop. Diuretics are also employed to lower blood pressure and they are believed to act by dilating small arteries.

Efforts to control or prevent hypertension by altering diet have been tried. The high incidence of this disease has declined in Japan when people have been taken off their high salt diets. Sasaki of Hirosaki University, in observing a large series of cases, showed that high salt intake produces high blood pressure and strokes. Priddle and coworkers of Toronto have demonstrated the value of low sodium diets in treating hypertension. American physicians have also prescribed low salt and sodium diets for their hypertensive patients.

Chapter Twelve

GASTROINTESTINAL DRUGS

THE DIGESTIVE TRACT begins with the intake of food in the mouth and ends at the anus or outlet of the rectum where feces are extruded. In between, marvelous chemical processes take place in which foods are broken down into basic components for absorption into the body. All portions of this wonderously conceived system are subject to disease.

The mouth and throat are vulnerable to virus and bacterial infections. Treatment is similar to that of the respiratory tract. Teeth are also susceptible to disease, and the dentist takes care of this portion of the anatomy. Occasionally, there is difficulty in swallowing. This may be on a purely nervous basis or it may be due to organic disease.

As food leaves the throat and moves down the esophagus, it comes to the stomach. This organ's function is very easily upset by irritating foods, nervousness and emotional upheavals. The stomach also reacts to disorders elsewhere in the body.

ACUTE GASTRITIS

Acute gastritis is an inflammation of the stomach. It may be produced by dietary indiscretion, alcohol, infectious diseases, ingestion of corrosive substances, and other causes. Treatment is directed towards the inciting factor. The diagnosis is made from the history or from direct examination of the stomach through an instrument known as the gastroscope. Symptoms may be mild or severe and consist of pain in the stomach, soreness, heartburn, fullness, nausea, vomiting, belching, and passing of gas by rectum.

If the condition is mild, food is restricted temporarily to bland substances. Together with an antacid, this may be enough to achieve relief. If severe, and vomiting is part of the picture, fluids will have to be given intravenously to replace the loss. Compazine® and Tigan® are usually effective in halting vomiting. Compazine® is tranquilizing, too. These drugs can be given by injection or rectal suppositories. When nausea and vomiting cease, then antacids may be administered orally. When bacterial infection exists, then antibiotics are indicated. In patients who have ingested corrosive substances, lavage (washing out) of the stomach is necessary and antidotes for the poisons are given. Soothing preparations such as aluminum gel can be taken orally. Narcotics for pain, and intravenous fluids to make up fluid loss by vomiting, may be prescribed.

EXCESSIVE GAS

Normally there are about 100 to 150 cubic centimeters of air in the stomach or intestine at any one time, and an individual ordinarily passes between 1000 and 1500 cubic centimeters of odorless gas (flatus) each day. Flatulence, or gaseous bloating, may be bothersome and results in symptoms of belching, stomach and/or intestinal distension, abdominal pain, and rumbling in the bowel (borborygmi).

There are a number of reasons for this disorder such as nervous tension with excessive swallowing of air, excessive formation of carbon dioxide in the colon because of failure of absorption or rapid small-intestinal motility, formation of excessive methane, hydrogen, and hydrogen sulfide by intestinal bacteria, and lack of hydrochloric acid in the stomach.

The nervous patient must be cautioned about his air swallowing problem and, if need be, he may be given sedatives or tranquilizers.

Certain bacteria in the bowel form gas and can be controlled with non-absorbable sulfa drugs such as Sulfathalidine® and Sulfasuxidine®, or Entero-Vioform®, or the tetracyclines. A common food they ferment into gas is the well-known bean. If the stomach lacks the normal quantity of hydrochloric acid (achlorhydria or hypoacidity), the ordinary intestinal bacteria will multiply and abnormal organisms will appear, also, to increase fermentation and gas volume. Antibiotics, ingestion of dilute hydrochloric acid or Acidulin® with meals, or the taking of Lactobacillus (Bacid® or Lactinex®) to reduce the activity of the normal bacterial flora, should ameliorate the problem. Sometimes hyperacidity, in ulcer patients, may result in gaseousness and is treated accordingly.

Elderly patients, who have a poorly functioning colon, complain frequently of distension. Poor digestion of foods leads to increasing fermentation and production of gas. Loss of tone slows intestinal movement producing further stasis. Constipation is best treated with a low carbohydrate diet, increased fluid intake, some exercise, and stool softeners such as Metamucil® or Dulcolax®, a very gentle laxative.

DIARRHEA

Diarrhea is an evacuation of watery or loose stools. It may be a primary disorder caused by extreme nervousness or fear, food sensitivity or poisoning, drugs, infection, and allergy, or it may be secondary to some other disease.

Symptoms are variable and may be quite minor or, on the other hand, severe with abdominal pain, nausea, vomiting, and frequent loose or watery stools. The attack may be of short duration or last for many days. Severe cases may develop dehydration, exhaustion, toxemia, collapse, and even death. Cholera is such an example. Mild cases of diarrhea will require no treatment. Severe cases may need fluids intravenously to combat dehydration. For cramping pains atropine can be given by injection. Donnagel® contains antipasmodics and coating medications. Neomycin® is also combined with Donnagel® for its antibiotic properties. Compazine® or Thorazine® will stop vomiting. Opiates are administered for severe pain and to slow down excessive intestinal motility. Lomotil® is also of value for these conditions. Paregoric is a well known opiate remedy and may be prescribed orally, if there is no vomiting.

Among the soothing agents employed for diarrhea are kaolin, pectin, bismuth, and aluminum hydroxide gel. Intestinal antiseptics are the non-absorbable Sulfasuxidine® and Sulfathalidine®, neomycin, Furoxone®, and the tetracyclines. In cases of staphylococcic food poisoning, the tetracyclines or the erythromycins may be effective. If the patient goes into shock, appropriate shock treatment will be ordered.

PEPTIC ULCER

Emotional stress plays an important role in causing peptic ulcer, but certain drugs such as aspirin, Butazolidine®, indomethacin, and the corticosteroids can induce ulcer formation. At least 10% of people have had the condition at some time during their lives according to autopsy reports. It does not occur when hydrochloric acid is absent in the stomach. It is common when there is hyperacidity. Stress and strain stimulate excessive acid production in the stomach. The usual sites of peptic ulcer are the stomach or just beyond it in the duodenum. The diagnosis is made by history, the finding of hyperacidity, x-rays, and, if necessary, by direct gastroscopic examination.

Pain is the outstanding symptom and it may be gnawing, burning, or aching in character. It occurs in rhythmic fashion with the intake of food, being relieved by food when duodenal, and intensified when a gastric ulcer. The complications of peptic ulcer are hemorrhages and perforations.

Treatment is usually medical, and, if this regimen fails, then surgery is considered. As most of the victims are under emotional stress, sedatives or tranquilizers are indicated. Formerly, to reduce hyperacidity, sodium bicarbonate and Sippy powders were prescribed, and also frequent ingestion of milk and cream. Milk is still used, but cream is now omitted, because it increases the cholesterol values of the blood. Antacids, such as Creamalin®, Maalox®, Gelusil®, and Amphojel®, are prescribed to lower hyperacidity, and this is important to achieve healing. Smoking should be avoided also.

Diet is not effective, as formerly believed, to heal ulcers. However, certain substances will aggravate ulcer symptoms such as condiments, alcohol, and coffee. Antispasmodic drugs decrease gastric secretion and motility. Among those employed in ulcer therapy are atropine, belladonna, Daricon®, Pathilon®, Probanthine®, Lomotil®.

ULCERATIVE COLITIS

This disorder frequently reflects emotional storms. Many of these patients are immature, tense, hostile, and hypersensitive. but outwardly are timid and submissive. Psychotherapy along with medical therapy is more successful than either one alone.

There are also non-psychiatric factors in ulcerative colitis. Certain foods may play an irritative role, and this is especially true when the colon is allergic to specific foods. If they are omitted from the diet, there is often a dramatic recovery. Carbohydrate or gluten intolerance by the colon may produce ulcerative colitis. Surgical removal of part of the stomach may result in carbohydrates provoking the colon.

When the colon is very irritable, the diet may have to be restricted to avoid any food or drink that stimulates evacuation. Low residue foods are also indicated. Vitamin deficiencies must be avoided. Antimicrobial therapy is given and includes such drugs as the tetracyclines, Asulfidine® Sulfasuxidine®, Sulfathalidine®, or other sulfa drugs, and even penicillin. Antispasmodics, antidiarrheics, and tranquilizers are employed. Where there is extreme fluid loss, intravenous feedings will be given. In cases of marked hemorrhages, blood plasma, red blood cells, or blood will be administered. The corticosteroids are sometimes very valuable, especially if there is associated allergy. Surgery is employed to stop massive hemorrhages or to treat bowel perforation resulting in peritonitis.

IRRITABLE COLON

Irritable colon is also known as spastic colon and mucous colitis. The disorder signifies a disturbance in colon function as the result of emotional tension and stress, and constitutes up to 50% of gastrointestinal disorders.

Symptoms are abdominal pain, fullness, discomfort after eating, gaseous distensions, passing of gas by rectum (flatus), diarrhea of varying degrees accompanied by mucus and small stools, periods of constipation, nausea, belching, fatigue, shortness of breath, and headache. The onset of the condition coincides with periods of emotional stress, and these neurotic people fight their conflicts in their colons. When the situations resolve, the disorder quiets down. But if problems again arise, another attack of the irritable colon syndrome may be expected.

Treatment consists of psychotherapy, tranquilizers or sedatives, and antispasmodics. If the patient is having a diarrheal or constipation episode appropriate treatment should be given.

CONSTIPATION

Perhaps one of the greatest obsessions in the USA is bowel

fixation, and of course this means constipation. Some people feel that one hard movement a day is constipation, while others believe it is the failure of daily evacuation. Vast sums of money are spent in advertising laxatives, and this is a very lucrative business, for Americans are very bowel conscious. The essential function of the colon, when it receives the liquid contents of the small intestine, is to absorb the water and form a fecal mass for evacuation. When the process is finished and ready for extrusion, the mass is moved into the rectum where the urge to defecate arises.

Some people have a bowel movement every day, others every two or three days, a few even longer. So the interval varies with each individual, and should not be upset with laxatives. Some people are constipated because they do not drink enough fluids, and, if the liquid intake is increased, constipation is alleviated. Taking a large glass of warm water upon arising, flavored with some fruit juice to be palatable, will very often be effective. More fluids can be taken with or after breakfast. A definite time, preferably after breakfast, for sitting on the toilet, should be tried. Once rhythm is established, the problem is under control.

For those who have lost the urge to go, a simple enema routine may be effective in starting a rhythm. If this proves insufficient, then bulk formers such as Metamucil®, Cellothyl®, or methylcellulose may be prescribed. Laxatives are sometimes used by patients who get discouraged, but cathartics are merely whipping boys for the intestine.

A few other items should be considered. It is essential that older patients have a full complement of hydrochloric acid in their stomachs. If it is greatly diminished or absent, hydrochloric acid may be administered in dilute form or as Acidulin® capsules. A diet rich in vitamin B stimulates intestinal motility. Lactic-acid bacteria in the bowel impedes the growth of the putrefactive organisms. They may be supplied by yogurt, acidophilus milk, or acidophilus cultures. Milk furnishes the lactose needed for sustenance by these bacteria.

DIVERTICULOSIS OF THE COLON

Diverticuli of the colon are outpocketings in the bowel, occurring in areas where the wall has weakened. This condition is seen mostly after the age of 40, and it increases in frequency until, at the age of 80, about 50% of people have diverticuli.

A good many individuals with this disorder have no symptoms and require no treatment, although they are advised to eat a diet low in roughage, drink an adequate amount of liquids, and use a bulk forming agent such as Metamucil®. When the diverticuli become inflamed there is pain over the affected area, diarrhea or constipation or alternation of the two, and mucous or bloody discharge. Medical treatment consists of bed rest, fluids orally or intravenously, antibiotics for infection, medication for pain. Complications are obstruction or perforation of the bowel, and severe hemorrhage, all of which may require surgery.

ACUTE HEPATITIS

Acute hepatitis is an acute infection of the liver caused by a virus. Symptoms of the illness are fever, nausea, vomiting, abdominal distress, itching, jaundice, dark urine (because of bile appearing in it), and light stools (because of bile not getting into the bowel due to liver obstruction).

As there is no drug which will kill the virus, treatment is supportative. If the patient cannot take liquids orally, intravenous fluids must be given. A simple nourishing diet, high in vitamin content, is indicated if the patient is not vomiting. Albumin may be given intravenously if the liver is not producing enough to keep up the albumin blood level. Atropine or belladonna is advocated for nausea and heartburn. The liver is a detoxifier and so one must be careful in administering drugs which it may not be able to handle at this time.

GALL BLADDER DISEASE

Acute gall bladder inflammation (acute cholecystitis) is an acute infection of the gall bladder by microorganisms living in the intestine. Symptoms consist of indigestion and moderate to severe discomfort or pain in the right upper abdomen. Jaundice with dark colored urine may or may not be present.

For relief of pain, Demerol® or morphine combined with atropine may be utilized. Antispasmodics also reduce pain. Polycillin® (ampicillin) or the broad spectrum antibiotics are suggested for infection. Intravenous fluids may be given in order to rest the gastrointestinal tract and gall bladder. The gall bladder attack may last for several hours or for days. Complications are perforation or rupture of the gall bladder. Surgery may be needed to terminate the disease or to treat the complications.

Gall bladder stones (cholelithiasis) are found in 10 to 20% of adults, with the incidence rising in middle life. At the age of 75 years 1 out of 3 people have stones in the gall bladder.

The disorder may be absolutely symptomless or the patient may have vague feelings of fullness in the abdomen. If the stones obstruct the cystic duct leading out of the gall bladder or the bile duct from the liver to the intestine, the pain is very severe. It is located in the right upper portion of the abdomen, frequently radiating to the right shoulder.

For relief of pain morphine, Demerol®, atropine or other antispasmodics are employed. The cure of the disorder is surgical removal of the gall bladder.

CIRRHOSIS OF THE LIVER

Cirrhosis is a chronic liver disease which terminates in fibrosis or scarring of the liver. There are several types of cirrhosis. Laenec's cirrhosis, also called alcoholic or nutritional cirrhosis, is very common. Both alcohol and poor diet contribute to the disorder, and it can be prevented by avoiding alcohol and ingesting a diet rich in vitamins and proteins. Various infections and parasites damage the liver, and also chemical poisons in industry. A third type of cirrhosis is partial or complete obstruction of the bile carrying ducts of the liver caused by drugs or viruses.

Mild asymptomatic cirrhosis needs no therapy, but the patient should be on a very nutritious diet, avoid alcohol, and refrain from using liver damaging drugs or working with industrial poisons. The onset of symptoms is insidious. There is loss of appetite and weight, nausea, vomiting, fullness of the abdomen, jaundice, swelling of the abdomen with fluid (ascites), swelling of the legs, shallow breathing (because the fluid in the abdomen pushes the diaphragm up), and gradual general deterioration.

In advanced cases, a good nutritious diet with high vitamin content is advocated; sodium and salt intake should be reduced. Corticosteroids are of some value in reducing jaundice and improving appetite in biliary or toxic cirrhosis. Diuretics may be used to relieve the swelling of the abdomen and legs. Abdominal tapping is also prescribed to remove abdominal fluid. Esophageal varices or dilated veins caused by back pressure from the cirrhosis may rupture and call for surgical procedures.

HEMORRHOIDS

Most adults have hemorrhoids. These veins may cause no symptoms, may only prolapse and be easily replaced in the rectum, or they may cause trouble. If these veins become swollen and thrombosed (clotted), so that they cannot be replaced, and if they become ulcerated or infected, or hemorrhage, then we have an uncomfortable patient.

Mildly irritated hemorrhoids are treated with medicated suppositories to provide relief and shrinking. Constipation should be avoided as it aggravates the condition. Massively swollen prolapsed hemorrhoids are treated with cooling solutions, corticosteroids, injections of the local anesthetic Xylocaine® and the enzyme Wydase® to reduce swelling. Then the patient may elect surgery. If there is some tissue death (necrosis) of the hemorrhoids, they may be treated with hot compresses and pain relieving agents, later followed by surgery. Treatment for hemorrhoids is either injection of sclerosing (scarring) agents or surgical amputation.

Chapter Thirteen

SKIN AND ALLERGY DRUGS

ALLERGY WAS DEFINED in 1906 by von Pirquet, coiner of the name, as an altered reaction to the entrance of a foreign substance. The normal individual, for example, does not react to pollen, but the allergic person responds to such intrusion with hay fever.

An antigen is an inciting material which causes the formation of an allergic antibody. An allergen was formerly defined as a substance producing allergy, probably forming an antibody, but the latter was not definitely confirmed. However, the terms allergen and antigen are now interchangeable in common usage.

Allergic disease is constantly increasing. Formerly one person in ten suffered from this disorder, but new government figures say one in seven is afflicted. This means that 31,000,000 Americans are affected, and 3 out of 4 suffer from hay fever and/or asthma. According to the claim of the American Allergy Foundation, allergies are No. 1 in terms of the number of people in the USA afflicted by any disease.

All systems of the body are subject to allergic disorders. Commonly recognized by the layman are asthma, hay fever, migraine, eczema, drugs like penicillin, horse serum, food and cosmetic allergy. But he is not so aware of allergy of the joints, nervous system, cardiovascular and urinary systems, nose and sinuses, eye, blood, and gastrointestinal system.

Allergens may be things we eat, inhale, touch, are injected with, or infected by. In addition, breakdown products or new chemical compounds formed in our bodies by interactions with infectants, inhalants, ingestants, or drugs, also create new allergens. Consequently, the increasing number of new chemical products each year, plus the enormous number of pollutants, makes us constantly vulnerable to increasing numbers of new allergens. That we survive is a miracle of endurance.

BRONCHIAL ASTHMA

Bronchial asthma is a disease in which the bronchial tubes go into spasm, thus reducing the amount of air going into the lungs. It may be produced by allergy or irritating substances. Allergens which may trigger these attacks are pollens, molds, dusts, mites, drugs, foods, animal products, infections, and miscellaneous agents. Nonallergic items are emotions, odors, heat or cold, air pollution, overactivity, and atmospheric conditions.

Symptoms are shortness of breath, wheezing, coughing with raising of very thick mucus, pallor, anxiety, fear of strangling, and cyanosis (blueness from lack of oxygen).

The acute attack of bronchial asthma is relieved by injections of adrenalin or orally administered ephedrine. Opiates are not given as they inteisify bronchial tube obstruction, but Demerol® does not have this property. The latter may be used or the tranquilizers to give the patient rest. Oxygen is employed to reduce cyanosis. Expectorants, like potassium iodide or ammonium chloride, loosen the thick mucus plugs in the bronchial tubes. When adrenalin or ephedrine is ineffective, aminophylline is administered intravenously, by rectal enema or rectal suppository.

If infection is triggering the attack antibiotics are prescribed. Frequently, asthmatics are dehydrated and fluids must be given either by mouth or intravenously, otherwise the mucus becomes very thick and tenacious, and very difficult to raise. Enzymes are sometimes used in aerosols to split the mucus. Corticosteroids are of value in relieving asthma.

Therapy should be directed to forestalling future attacks. Allergens should be avoided when possible, and if not, the patient should receive hyposensitizing injections to the offending agent whenever possible. An allergic workup with tests and analysis of the patient and his environment is needed, so that proper advice and treatment is rendered to forestall future attacks.

NASAL ALLERGY AND HAY FEVER

While allergic bronchial asthma is a sensitivity of the lower respiratory tract, nasal allergy involves the upper portion of the tract. Actually the allergy, many times, starts in the nose and sinuses and then spreads downward to the bronchial tubes or the course of action may be reversed. Then again, allergy may strike the entire tract at about the same time.

Seasonal nasal allergy (allergic rhinitis) is also known as hay fever, because originally the malady was thought to be due to hay. This erroneous conception was eventually noted, but the name still stuck. Hay fever occurs at specific times of the year when molds, tree, grass, and ragweed pollens are airborn. Then there is also the year around nasal allergy due to foods, feathers, animal danders, drugs, house dust, mites, inhalants, infections, and other agents.

Symptoms of nasal allergy are sneezing, nasal discharge and blockage, headaches, itching of the nose, eyes, and throat. The nasal and sinus membranes are swollen from the reaction between allergen and antibody, and they discharge mucus which floods the nose and runs down into the throat producing a cough. In the allergic reaction, histamine is liberated along with other cellular breakdown products. For allergic responses damage tissues. Secondary infection may be superimposed upon the allergic condition.

Effective in relieving the nasal symptoms are the antihistamines, ephedrine, or Sudafed® (a pseudoephedrine). Drugs like Triaminic®, Dimetapp®, Co-Pyronil®, and Naldecon® contain antihistamines and constrictors to reduce nasal swelling. Nasal sprays containing constrictors are also available. Corticosteroids may give prolonged relief by blocking the inflammation. One such product is Turbinaire®, available as a nasal medication.

Preventive treatment is possible by getting a good history, performing allergy tests to determine the offenders, and hyposensitizing the patients with allergy vaccines. Sometimes the patient deliberately leaves his environment and takes a vacation during the hay fever season. Molds, however, are ubiquitous and hyposensitizing is recommended. Infections are treated with antibiotics. An allergic profile of the patient enables the physician to advise the patient how to avoid exposure, the measures to be taken, and the antiallergic treatment needed.

DRUG ALLERGY

Adverse drug reactions are either allergic or nonallergic. The nonallergic response consists of unwanted side reactions, toxic effects, intolerance, idiosyncrasy, and interreactions.

Drug allergies are similar in their responses to other allergens. They give rise to fever, hives (urticaria), joint pain and swelling, and enlargement of lymph nodes or glands, as in horse serum allergy. A severe allergic reaction, known as anaphylaxis, is characterized by nausea, vomiting, shortness of breath, wheezing, pulmonary edema (lung swelling), fever, cyanosis, and even shock. The individual may die very quickly unless medical care is given, as exemplified in penicillin allergic reactions. Drug allergy may involve the nervous system and brain, cardiovascular system, respiratory tract, gastrointestinal system, kidney system, blood, connective tissue components, and skin.

In treating severe reactions, which may be life threatening, the physician may use adrenalin, antihistamines, corticosteroids, and aminophylline. Shock measures may be also utilized. For less severe reactions antihistamines or corticosteroids can be employed. Substitution of a nonallergic drug will be mandatory for treating whatever disease the patient has.

ALLERGY TO INSECT STINGS

Individuals may develop allergy to insect stings or bites, the most dramatic being those due to wasps, bees, and hornets. For, if the person who is stung is very sensitive to the venom, death may ensue almost immediately. Adrenalin is the emergency drug for saving a life in this circumstance. Antihistamines are also valuable and so are the corticosteroids, and they may be used concomitantly. If the reaction is not severe, the latter two drugs may be administered orally along with ephedrine when the physician so judges.

Local treatment is designed to remove the venom sac of the bee carefully. This is done by scraping off the sac with the finger or a knife, not by grasping it, for more venom may be injected by this action. Ice packs may be applied to the sting area.

Hyposensitization is carried out by using injections of the particular insect venom to which the individual is very allergic. This treatment will often prove to be life-saving when the person is stung again, for there will be either very little or no reaction to the sting. It is also a good idea for persons prone to stings of bees, wasps, and hornets to carry a specially prepared kit for use in such emergencies.

ALLERGIC SKIN DISEASES

Skin allergies are very common and make up a large proportion of skin diseases. The most outstanding are urticaria (hives), atopic dermatitis (allergic eczema), and contact dermatitis.

Urticaria (Hives) is very familiar to most people. It is characterized by itching wheals on the body. If severe, and the wheals coalescence to form gigantic hives (angioedema), one may observe marked swelling of the lips, face, and throat. Massive swelling in the throat may cause an individual to strangle, unless emergency medical care is available. Adrenalin will usually reduce the swelling quickly, and this may be reinforced by antihistamines and corticosteroids. If time is of the essence, it may be necessary to do a tracheotomy (make an opening into the windpipe) to prevent strangulation.

Usually, antihistamines or ephedrine by mouth are sufficient to provide relief from hives. One should, however, search for the allergens responsible for causing the attack. They are usually foods, drugs, or infections. Elimination or hyposensitization is in order. It should be emphasized that all cases of hives are not necessarily allergic.

Atopic Dermatitis (Allergic Eczema) usually starts in infancy and is initiated with food and/or inhalant allergies. This disorder coexists frequently with asthma, hay fever and nasal allergy. The eruptions occur on the face, neck, elbows and back of the knees. It is a weeping eczema in childhood and in later years becomes a dry, scaling, itchy rash.

Treatment consists of eliminating the allergens when possible. If not, hyposensitization is recommended. Local therapy may be wet dressings, or a steroid ointment or cream. Nonirritating soaps or cleansing agents are recommend such as Lowila®, Aveeno-Bar®, or Oilatum®. The skin is excessively dry and needs hydration. Baths with colloidal Aveeno®, Alpha Keri®, Lubath® or similar preparations are advocated. Local moisturizing agents are water, Nivea®, Keri® lotion or cream, Lubriderm®, Nutraspa®, Domol®, or similar agents.

Antihistamines are of value in controlling itching. Temaril® provides relief from itching, but may make the patient drowsy. If corticosteroids are needed, they are given for a short time by mouth or injection to get the patient "over the hump."

Contact Dermatitis is the most common skin disease and will remain in first place for many years to come. As more chemical products are produced each year, the chances for more cases of contact dermatitis increase. The condition is due to irritating or allergy producing substances getting on the skin. The list of items which can cause this disorder are legion. Common offenders are poison ivy and oak, cosmetics, drugs, industrial oils and chemicals, certain occupational hazards, resins, fabrics, enzymes, insecticides, detergents, soaps, fertilizers, paints, foods, and sprays.

At the area of contact, the skin becomes red, itchy, blistery, and weeping. The dermatitis may extend beyond this point by further contact or allergy. The first object of therapy is to remove the offending agent when known. Wet compresses may be applied, and, if the disease has become generalized, colloidal oatmeal (Aveeno®) baths will provide comfort and relief from itching. Corticosteroids may be given orally, topically, or by injection to provide relief from itching and reduce inflammation. Antihistamines are also helpful in allaying itching. Antibiotics are used for infection, when present.

In some cases, such as poison ivy or poison oak, hyposensitizing injections can be given for protection against future attacks. In other situations hyposensitizing procedures are not available and avoidance is the only possibility. A patient's skin may become immune to further insults by allergens, in some occupations, by what is called "hardening" of the skin. In other individuals this cannot be accomplished.

PSORIASIS

Psoriasis is a chronic thick-scaly disorder affecting usually the scalp, elbows, and knees, but may attack any part of the body including the face. The disease may be associated with arthritis. The cause is not known, but some ascribe an allergic background to it. Flareups are associated with emotional hangups and crises, infections, and other disturbances to body homeostasis.

Exposure of the skin to sunlight is often helpful, but in severe cases it may not work. Sedative or tranquilizers can be used to calm the patient when emotional problems are paramount.

Typical therapy consists in the application of drugs such as tar, salicylic acid, ammoniated mercury, or steroids. Tar and ultraviolet radiation have been a long standing effective procedure. Scalp psoriasis may be very stubborn to treat. Preparations used for this purpose are Alphosyl® shampoo, Baker's P & S liquid®, tar shampoos, and salicylic acid.

WARTS

Warts are caused by a virus. Usually, the body will develop an immunity and the warts disappear spontaneously. Some authorities have even claimed that psychotherapy will cause them to go. However, there are stubborn cases that will not yield to magic incantations. For these, several types of therapy are available such as acids, electrodestruction, and freezing with carbon dioxide or liquid nitrogen.

HERPES ZOSTER (SHINGLES)

Herpes is a virus disease which affects the skin. There seems to be a definite relationship between the herpes virus and the chicken pox virus, in fact some investigators think they are the same.

Shingles is characterized by marked pain on the involved side of the body, and crops of blister, on a red base, occur along the line of reaction. Analgesics or narcotics are given to relieve pain. Soothing remedies are applied to the skin. The corticosteroids may or may not be given locally or orally depending upon the judgement of the physician.

ACNE

Acne is the curse of youth. It is a disease with deep psychological impact, because of its unsightly appearance and scarring. Acne may be mild and consist mostly of whiteheads and blackheads, or on the other hand it may be accompanied by marked inflammation, infection, and abscesses.

Treatment consists of mechanical removel of the blackheads and whiteheads which plug ducts of the sebaceous or oil glands. If this is done properly, then the ducts will not rupture and pour their irritating contents into the adjacent tissue, thereby causing inflammation and infection that leads to scarring.

Cleansing agents with mild peeling properties are prescribed such as Acnaveen Bar®, Brasivol Scrub Cleaner®, Pernox®, Fostex Soap®, Acne-Aid Detergent Soap®.

Topically, acne medications are drugs such as benzoyl peroxide, corticosteroids, resorcinol and sulfur. Preparations available for this purpose are Benoxyl Lotion®, Fostril Cream®, Rezamin Lo-Vanoxide Lotion®, Liquimat®, Komed Lotion® and Cream®, Acnomel Cream®, and Acne-Dome Cream®. Ultraviolet radiation and carbon dioxide slush provide deeper peeling. Vitamin A is utilized to help prevent plugging of the openings of the ducts, vitamin A acid to provide more effective peeling of blackheads and whiteheads.

Infection in acne is mostly due to the Corynebacterium acnes organism, but the staphylococcus also is a factor. The tetracyclines are effective antibiotics in curbing acne infection.

It is generally believed that the male sex hormone (androgen) and the female hormone (progesterone) incite acne. The female estrogenic hormones neutralize the actions of these drugs and suppress the excessive oil flow on the skin, thereby improving acne. Grenz-ray radiation is helpful in reducing inflammation and excessive oil flow. X-ray is a more powerful agent on the skin and is used much less today.

Hypertrophic or built-up scarring can be improved by steroid injections which shrink the scar tissue. "Ice pick" scars may be removed by a circular punch or the scalpel (knife). Some scars can be surgically excised. Chemexfoliation (chemosurgery) improves shallow scars and gives the face a better appearance by providing a new skin surface. This method employs various drugs such as phenol, trichloracetic acid, or various modifications.

SKIN INFECTIONS

Skin infections are produced by viruses, bacteria, and fungi. These disorders may be localized or widespread. Antibiotics, chemotherapeutic agents, and chemical agents to combat and destroy these microorganisms are discussed in Chapter 6 of this book and the reader is referred back to this section if he wishes to review **the subject.**

Chapter Fourteen

ARTHRITIS DRUGS

THERE ARE A NUMBER of different types of arthritis such as traumatic, gouty, infectious, rheumatoid, and osteoarthritis.

TRAUMATIC ARTHRITIS

Traumatic arthritis is caused by injury which may damage any or all the anatomical parts of the joint. Treatment may be medical or surgical depending upon the nature and extent of the tearing and crushing. Medical treatment of arthritis will be discussed with other types of arthritis.

GOUTY ARTHRITIS

Gout is either a primary genetic defect in metabolism, or a secondary alteration of metabolism produced by blood disorders, starvation, obesity, cancer, alcoholism, cardiovascular and kidney disease, or other maladies. In gouty artritis, urate crystals are deposited in the joints. This brings on swelling and sometimes excruciating pain. Diagnosis is made by finding abnormal levels of uric acid in the blood.

During an acute attack of gouty arthritis, the drug of choice since ancient times has been colchicine. This medication may be used also in small doses to prevent recurrences. It is toxic and provokes nausea, vomiting, and severe diarrhea. The drug is stopped either when relief is obtained or diarrhea sets in. Other drugs used in acute attacks are the corticosteroids, Indocin® (indomethacin), and Butazolidin® (phenylbutazone).

Following the acute attack of gouty arthritis, one of several drugs may be prescribed to lower uric acid levels in the blood and prevent new attacks. Such preparations are Zyloprim® (allorpurinol), Benemid® (probenecid), and Anturan® (sulfinpyrazone). Patients are advised to use a diet low in purines, and to especially avoid foods like brains, liver, and sweetbreads. Alcohol should be avoided or consumed in small quantities.

INFECTIOUS ARTHRITIS

In infectious arthritis, the invading organisms are frequently found in the joints. This situation may occur in viral and bacterial disease. Gonorrheal organisms are often elicited from aspiration of joint fluid in patients with active gonorrhea showing signs of arthritis. The most common microorganisms found in infectious arthritis are the streptococcus, staphylococcus, meningococcus (meningitis), and pneumococcus. Diseases which may be accompanied by arthritis are tuberculosis, syphilis, German measles, brucellosis, typhoid fever, rheumatic fever, bacillary dysentery, and fungus disorders such as coccidioidomycosis, histoplasmosis, and actinomycosis. Treatment of the arthritis is the treatment of the primary source of the infection in the body. Drugs utilized for fighting these diseases are given in Chapter 6.

RHEUMATOID ARTHRITIS (ATROPHIC ARTHRITIS)

Three percent of the adult population of the USA suffers from rheumatoid arthritis. This malady is a chronic crippling illness. It attacks mostly the young, particularly females, and reaches its peak incidence between 30 to 50 years of age.

The course of the disease is variable. It may be mild with occasional remissions and relapses. On the other hand it may progress relentlessly, destroying and twisting the joints out of shape, and leaving the individual a stiff immobile cripple. The cause of the disease has not been generally settled, but allergists believe it to be an allergy, principally incited by infection somewhere in the body. In any event, rheumatoid arthritis is a systemic disorder, not just confined to the joints.

Early in the disease there is inflammation of one or more joints.

Later there is more involvement. Scar tissue forms and the joints become deformed. Hard nodules or lumps occur under the skin in about 25% of afflicted persons. There is also inflammation of arteries which may become quite diffuse. Certain changes are found in the blood, including a so-called rheumatoid factor.

Symptoms vary, depending upon the severity of the disease and the stage of development. The individual may date his initial symptoms from an acute episode such as a cold, sore throat, sinus attack, or other infection. The onset is often insidious. One or more joints are involved at the beginning, with stiffness being the most common complaint. Pain is noted mostly in severe inflammation. However, pain is produced by twisting movements of the hands and wrists, and occurs in the knees and feet when standing. There may or may not be a low grade fever, weakness, loss of appetite, and general fatigue.

The onset of the disease may be more spectacular with high fever, chills, multiple joint involvement, and a great deal of malaise. Sometimes rheumatoid arthritis smolders along for years without too much destruction, but eventually the ravages of the illness become apparent in the swelling of the fingers, wrists, hand, elbows, knees, ankles and other joints, along with stiffness, deformity, and loss of function.

Other systems frequently show pathologic changes. The spleen occasionally enlarges. Nodules and scarring may develop in the lungs. The kidneys may become affected. Anemia is noted. In 3 to 5% of persons there is eye inflammation sometimes during the course of the disease.

Treatment of rheumatoid arthritis consists of general rest, with protection of afflicted joints but not necessarily absolute immobilization, for such a procedure could result in a stiff frozen joint. Deformities once acquired, are not easy to reverse. After recovery from an attack, reasonable exercise of the joints is indicated to prevent deformity.

Physical therapy, especially heat, has long been advocated. It may consist of hot packs, hot baths, hot soaks, or the Hubbard tank which permits both heat and exercise therapy.

The main drug used is aspirin, and this can be taken as such, or as Bufferin®, Ascriptin®, or any other preparation desired. Sodium salicylate has also been employed. Darvon® and codeine are used for relief of pain, if aspirin is not effective.

Other antiarthritic drugs are Butazolidin®, gold salts, corticosteroids, Indocin®, and antimalarial drugs. The corticosteroids may be given orally, by injection, or by direct introduction into a particular joint.

Antiallergic therapy consists in looking for allergens, especially the locales for visible or latent infections, with the hope of eradicating them. Hyposensitizing, if successful, may bring the disorder under control. Surgical therapy has advanced spectacularly in the last decade. Joints may be repaired or restored with prosthetics.

OSTEOARTHRITIS (DEGENERATIVE ARTHRITIS)

While rheumatoid arthritis is called the "arthritis of the young," osteroarthritis is the "arthritis of the aged." It is usually noted in middle life starting around the age of 50 and continuing on into old age. Osteoarthritis is the commonest type of arthritis. It is considered to be caused by wear and tear on the joints over the years, aging of the bone and cartilage in the joints, trauma, abnormal weight-bearing on the joints as in obesity. Low grade infection and infectious allergy through the years probably contributes to the eventual degeneration of the joints, although this is not mentioned as a factor.

The characteristics of this condition are the destruction of the cartilage and overgrowth of the ends of the bones. Sites of involvement are the fingers, wrists, ankles, knees, hips, and shoulder joints, as well as the spine in the neck and lower back regions. There is often a lack of correlation between x-ray findings and symptoms. Sometimes the person with marked changes has little or no symptoms while another with minimal reaction has much discomfort. Aching pain is the common manifestation of this malady. It is rarely very intense and is relieved by resting the joint. A common finding, especially in women, is enlargement of the terminal finger joints. This is called Heberden's nodes.

Drug treatment for this disease is designed to relieve the aching pain. Aspirin or aspirin compounds, Tylenol®, and Darvon® provide analgesic action. Butazolidin®, Indocin®, and the corticosteroids are also administered. The latter is usually injected into painful joints.

Physical therapy employing heat in various forms, ultrasound, and exercises, are frequently utilized. Obesity must be reduced, if relief to weight-bearing joints is desired.

Orthopedic surgery is used where other measures have failed to provide relief from pain and reverse joint instability. Prostheses are introduced into the body when indicated.

Chapter Fifteen

URINARY TRACT DRUGS

THE URINARY TRACT becomes infected by direct invasion through the urethra, or by blood born bacteria.

ACUTE URETHRITIS

Acute urethritis is an inflammation of the urethra, the urinary passage leading from the bladder to the outside of the body. The female is more liable to infection than the male, because of contamination from adjacent structures and the shortness of her urethra.

In the male, gonorrhea is the chief cause of this inflammation. However, other disease-producing organisms may invade this structure. In the female the common pathogens are the colon bacillus and the gonorrheal microbe. Ordinarily, the symptoms consist of discomfort and burning on urination, backache, abdominal pain, fatigue, and possibly fever. For infection, penicillin or another antibiotic may be used. Urinary tract drugs, like Gantrisin® and Furadantin®, are frequently prescribed for urethritis. Pain relievers and antispasmodics are given for relief of discomfort until the infection is brought under control. At this time, the symptoms should have abated.

ACUTE CYSTITIS

Acute cystitis is an inflammation of the bladder, which occurs in both sexes. It may be incited by microbiotic invasion from the urethra or descending involvement from the kidneys. A common pathogen is the colon bacillus. In the male, enlargement of the prostate causes stasis of urine in the bladder and therapy contributes to infection.

In cystitis, the sufferers complain of pain on voiding, frequency of urination, discomfort in the bladder region, and possibly backache. Pus and blood is often noted in the urine. Bladder cancer can also mimic an ordinary cystitis. Drugs used for urethral discharge and prostatitis may be employed in cystitis. Additional drugs prescribed are mandelic acid and methanamine, which have been solely urinary tract medications for years. Antispasmodics may be ordered to ease the complaints of the patient until the specific drugs take effect.

ACUTE PROSTATITIS

Prostatitis is an inflammation of the prostate gland in men. It may be caused by gonorrhea or some other bacteria as the result of direct extension from the urethra, bladder, kidney, or blood stream.

There is frequently difficulty in voiding, backache, pelvic discomfort and sometimes fever. Pus may be observed in the urine. The choice of antibiotic depends upon the infecting organism. Commonly employed in the condition are penicillin, ampicillin, tetracyclines, Gantanol® and Furadantin®.

ACUTE GLOMERULONEPHRITIS (INFLAMED KIDNEYS)

Acute inflammation of the kidneys, known as acute glomerulonephritis, is an allergic reaction produced in these organs by a streptococcal infection elsewhere in the body. Such locales are usually in the tonsils, throat, and sinuses. The disorder frequently arises about 10 days to 2 weeks after such an infection. The initial signs of the kidney inflammation are blood in the urine, decrease of urine output, possibly some body swelling, an increase in blood pressure, fatigue and abnormal findings in the urine.

In treating this condition, sodium is usually restricted to reduce swelling and prevent or lower hypertension. Penicillin or erythromycin is used to control the streptococcal infection which may still be latent in the body. Rest and diet are very important too.

Heparin and immunosuppressive drugs are being tried to minimize acute kidney damage. If brain swelling appears as a complication of the kidney disease then magnesium sulfate or 50% glucose can be given intravenously to reduce the edema.

KIDNEY STONES

Kidney stone formation is not fully understood. Whatever the cause or causes, substances which should be in solution, precipitate out in the calyces or pelvis of the kidneys and a stone buildup ensues.

Some stones are silent residents and remain so in the kidneys for years. The presence of others evokes a dull pain in the flanks or back. Many stones are passed without discomfort. However, when a stone enters the ureter and obstructs it, then excruciating pain arises which usually requires a narcotic and/or an antispasmodic to bring relief. The stone may then pass. If not, surgery may be required. Large stones in the pelvis or calyces of the kidney often need surgical removal because of obstruction and damage to the kidney.

Chapter Sixteen

PARASITIC DRUGS

Parasites have plagued man continuously since his first appearance on earth, and animals are not spared either by these ubiquitous creatures.

PEDICULOSIS (LICE)

The louse has tormented man throughout recorded history. The most common varieties are the head louse, the body louse, and the pubic louse. They are greedy little blood-suckers. Lice attach their nits (eggs) to hairs or clothing fibers. The victim of their attack frequently becomes allergic to their saliva or feces, and it is this sensitization which produces the symptoms. Nonallergic individuals have no symptoms. The usual complaint is itching. The diagnosis is made by finding the nits or lice in the hair. The disease is acquired by contact with an infected person or his clothing.

Kwell® is the drug of choice for eradicating this disorder. Secondary infection from scratching is treated with antibiotics. Clothing should be sterilized. In mass delousing operations, Lindane® or DDT are blown into the clothing. The body louse can transmit typhus, trench fever and relapsing fever.

SCABIES (THE SEVEN YEAR ITCH)

The human itch mite (sarcoptes scabiei) causes scabies. Contact with an infected person, or his linen or clothing, may initiate the disease. The diagnosis is confirmed by finding the burrowing which the mites make in the skin. If the tunnels are opened, the organism can be scraped out and identified under the microscope.

Newly infected individuals have no symptoms. Nightly itching commences about 30 days after infection, because of the burrowing and the development of allergy to the mite and his products. Treatment consists of the application of Kwell® to the body. Clothing and bedding should be heat sterilized to prevent reinfection.

PULEX IRRITANTS (FLEAS)

The human flea, Pulex irritans, attacks animals as well as humans. In retribution, one might say, cat, dog and rat fleas readily attack man. The skin irritation begins when the host becomes allergic to the salivary secretions of these blood-sucking parasites. Flea bites occur in clusters or in linear fashion. Fleas transmit such diseases as bubonic plague, murine typhus, tularemia and dog tapeworm.

The parasites must be eliminated from the environment, in order for the host to be cured. Dogs and cats now have flea collars which are quite effective. Breeding places, such as cracks in the floors, the space under the rugs, furniture, resting places of pets and rubbish piles should be sprayed. Washing of clothing and other washables eradicates fleas from these materials. The bites are treated with topical preparations to relieve itching. Antibiotics are used for infection, and corticosteroids as needed.

NEMATODES (ROUNDWORMS)

It is estimated that well over 3 billion people in this world are infected with roundworms, flatworms and flukes.

Roundworms infest the intestinal tract. There may or may not be symptoms. These parasites may give rise to abdominal discomfort and pain, loss of appetite, fatigue, nervousness, anemia, skin rashes, generalized aches and pains. The diagnosis is confirmed by the passing and identification of the worm, or by finding the eggs or worms in the stool.

The ascaris variety of roundworm is eliminated with piperazine citrate. The whipworm repsonds to thiabendazole. Hookworms are treated with tetrachloroethylene or bephenium. Pinworms are eradicated with piperazine or pyrvinium pamoate. The worms of creeping eruption and trichinosis (found in raw pork) are killed by thiabendazole.

CESTODES (TAPEWORMS)

Tapeworms are parasites which live in the intestinal tract. They may cause no symptoms or the host may have abdominal aching or pains, diarrhea and nervousness. Anemia may also be present. Recognition of the disorder becomes apparent when the worm or the eggs are found in the stools. Beef and fish tapeworms infections are treated with niclosamide or quinacrine. The latter drug is also used against the pork tapeworm, while the former drug is given for the dwarf tapeworm. Prevention of the disease is accomplished by eating only cooked beef, fish, or pork.

TREMATODES (FLUKES)

Flukes are flatworms with external muscular suckers for attaching themselves to their host. The Chinese liver fluke (Clonorchis sinensis), is very prevalent in the Far East. Human infection is acquired by eating raw fish, which has been infested with the parasite. There may or may not be symptoms. The diagnosis is made from the history of eating raw fish, abdominal pains, enlarged liver, diarrhea, systemic toxicity and finding of the parasite. Chloroquine® and Hetol® are the most favored drugs for treating this condition. The lung fluke (Paragonimus westermani) is very widespread in the Orient. Infection is caused by eating infested crayfish or crabs, or drinking infested water. The worms invade the lungs and produce symptoms mimicking tuberculosis. The diagnosis is established by the history, the prevalence of the disease in a community, and finding the eggs of the parasite in the sputum or stool. Bithinonil® is the drug of choice for eliminating the disease.

The blood flukes (Schistosomes) migrate from the bowels into the blood circulation and reach the liver, lungs, and central nervous system. Next to malaria, infestation by the blood flukes is man's most serious and widespread infection. It is constantly increasing while malaria is decreasing. Because the organism becomes so widespread in the body, symptoms are quite variable. Drugs utilized for treating this disease are stibophen, antimony potassium tartrate and other antimony preparations.

Drugs, Demons, Doctors, and Disease

SCHISTOSOME DERMATITIS (SWIMMERS ITCH, CLAM DIGGER'S ITCH)

Swimmer's Itch is a world wide condition, also prevalent in the USA. It is caused by worms transmitted by snails which are infected by the droppings of migratory birds, ducks, and rodents also infected with schistosomes. Fresh water bathers often get this disease. It is also called Clam Digger's Itch and the marine form is found in sea bathers on both coasts of the USA. The schistosome invades the skin and its burrowing sites become very itchy. Scratching may lead to secondary infection.

Rubbing the skin hard with a towel, after bathing in potentially infested water, will remove most of the parasites. Anti-itching preparation will provide relief for the uncomfortable skin. Antibiotics are indicated for secondary infection. Destruction of snails around bathing beaches is necessary to wipe out the disease.

MALARIA

This disorder is caused by four different Plasmodium parasites. The disease has been discussed previously in the book. At one time quinine was the drug of choice for malaria. It may be still used today, but newer medications have mostly replaced it. Such drugs are chloroquine, primaquine, amodiaquine, pyrimethamine, sulfadiazine or dapsone.

Drugs given internally to combat parasites have variable degrees of toxicity. They must be used cautiously and the patients should be supervised by a physician.

Chapter Seventeen

CANCER DRUGS

Because of the aura of mystery and dread surrounding cancer, no other affliction is held in such mortal fear. To many, the word is a dire pronouncement of death, with agonizing suffering and a very painful demise. The word cancer comes from the Latin and means crab, and it is easy to associate the little animal's tearing into tissues as similar to the invasion of a malignancy. The stealthy way in which the disease starts, and the ignorance of the victim that the growth is eating away his vital tissues until too late, has given the word cancer a terrifying connotation in the minds of people. No part of the body is immune to the disease.

Cancer exacts its annual toll. Close to half a million Americans will die of the malady this year. Fifty million, out of 200 million Americans now alive and in good health, will eventually have cancer. This represents 1 out of 4 individuals. Two thirds of those afflicted will die, unless new methods of treatment are found.

Cancer, also called carcinoma, is not a single disease, but multiple disorders, developing for different reasons, and needing different therapies. Yet there is one thing all carcinomas have in common, they once were normal cells but are now wild-growing uncontrollable cells. Actually they are parasites. For they take nourishment from the blood and lymph, contribute nothing of value to the body, invade adjacent normal tissue, and produce a multitude of cancer cells which they spew into the blood and lymph circulation to establish more parasitic colonies.

Drugs, Demons, Doctors, and Disease

If there is any evidence of intelligence or purpose in this unrestrained growth on nature's part, it is not lucidly clear. For the tumor in destroying its host, also destroys itself. It is like the story of the lemmings running down to the sea, jumping in, swimming until exhausted, and then drowning. Therefore, if the host does not benefit from the malignancy, or the malignancy from itself, then one can only assume that nature created cancerous growths to kill off living forms so as to control population. Cancer, accordingly, is only another lethal disease. Man, in trying to find a cure for or control the disease, is attempting to thwart nature as he has in whipping other deadly diseases.

The baffling question about cancer is what happens to a cell to cause it to lose its delicately balanced control-mechanism and suddenly start a disorganized prolific growth. Normally the genes in the nucleus of the cell contain DNA (deoxyribonucleic acid) which produces RNA (ribonucleic acid). This latter substance moves out of the nucleus into the cytoplasm of the cell with encoded orders for controlling cellular metabolism. If some situation should arise to alter or damage DNA or RNA messenger, then orderly growth control could conceivably be lost. Slight variation might produce a benign tumor, while a more marked change might give rise to a malignant growth. Radiation, chemicals, and viruses presumably produce cancer in this fashion.

Viruses are actually nothing more than tiny strands of DNA or RNA enclosed in a protein protective coating. In causing cancer, as opposed to ordinary viral diseases, the viral DNA or RNA enters the cell and forces the cell to make cancerous DNA. The question that immediately arises is why we don't all develop cancer, especially when the same viruses presumably invade all our bodies in the course of a lifetime. The answer seems to be a breakdown in immunity, somewhere along the line of resistance.

The body somehow recognizes foreign cells, such as in transplants, and reacts against them. But it does not recognize its own cancer cells as being foreign. Yet experiments have been performed in which two dying cancer patients, with similar tumors, have had some of their cancer tissue transplanted into each other. After a suitable interval of time, the patients are injected with each other's lymphocytes, which are antibody-producing white cells. Their cancers reduce in size and some even disappear. Why cannot their own lymphocytes do the job?

It is known that many types of cancer cells have antigens which should stimulate their own body's lymphocytes to produce antibodies to destroy these cancer cells. Yet they do not. It is postulated that cancer cells in some way protect or wall off their antigenic sites against their host's defensive mechanism, a sort of primitive instinct of self preservation. Bacteria often envelop themselves in protective coatings to prevent the body's fighting cells and antibodies from reaching and destroying them. In cancer, the host's own cells are destroying the host and protecting themselves from a just reprisal. From a philosophic viewpoint, how similar is this to animal and human behavior!

Substances causing cancer are known as carcinogens. If these carcinoma-inciting agents can be avoided, many types of cancer can be prevented. The first recognized occupational cancer was noted in 1775 by Percival Pott in England, who observed that chimney sweepers developed scrotal cancer from constant contact with soot. In more modern times, occupationally related carcinomas have been associated with coal tar and its derivatives, lignite, oil, shale, petroleum, metals and radioactive ores, metallic compounds, asbestos and other substances. Also considered carcinogenic are agricultural chemicals such as pesticides, oral contraceptives, products of molds and fungi, cigars, cigarettes, pipe smoking, sunlight, x-ray, radium, viruses and products produced by environmental pollution.

Strange associations have been elicited between cancer and various substances. In the dyestuff industry, Rehn in 1895 noted a high incidence of bladder cancer in people working with aniline dyes. In 1954 and 1966, Case showed the carcinogen was not the aniline but aromatic amine contaminants. Certain azo dyes used as food additives, especially butter yellow, were shown by Kinosita in 1936 to be carcinogens. Hot maize porridge in Curacao is associated with cancer of the esophagus. A cigar, made of tree bark and tobacco, and smoked in Thailand is believed to cause cancer of the larynx. The mold aspergillus, growing on corn, peanuts or cottonseed, produces aflatoxins which incite liver cancer. Cycasin, from the cyacad nut, produces cancer of the liver and kidney. Bladder cancer appeared in experimental animals when cyclamates were introduced into this organ.

LEUKEMIA

Leukemia is a malignancy of the white cells in which abnormal numbers are formed in the bone marrow or other sites. The disease is either acute or chronic, and there are three varieties of white cells involved in leukemia. They are lymphocytes, myelocytes, or monocytes. The type of leukemia is diagnosed by examining the blood and/or bone marrow.

Leukemia is believed to be caused by viruses. While radiation is associated with an increased incidence of leukemia, it may well be that the effects of radiation hasten the viral action. Symptoms in acute cases may come on quickly and usually consist of fever, prostration, bone or joint pain, bleeding from mucous membranes or into the skin, enlargement of lymph nodes, ulcertions of the mouth. However, symptoms may develop more slowly over a month or two with feelings of weakness, loss of appetite, fever and signs of an infection. In chronic cases, many times, the disease is diagnosed by a routine blood count. Frequently there are few or no pertinent signs. Patients may complain of enlarged lymph nodes, loss of appetite and weight, or an abdominal mass.

In 1970, Temin of Wisconsin, Baltimore of MIT, Gallo of the National Cancer Institute (NIC), along with Spiegelman of Columbia reported finding an enzyme called polymerase in leukemic patients. When these individuals are treated and undergoing remission, the enzyme decreases. During a relapse it rises again. A group of investigators at the NIC noted that a derivative of the antibiotic rifampicin, which is used to treat tuberculosis, blocks the RNA viral enzyme from forming cancerous DNA. Gallo believes that an antibody may be developed against this enzyme. Whether all human cancers are caused by viruses has not been fully determined.

In acute lymphocytic leukemia, a deadly disease in children, improvement is being achieved with a 4 drug combination, which results in increased survival time. The drugs are vincristine, prednisone (a corticosteroid), 6-mercaptopurine and methotrexate. Daunomycin, and a derivative called adriamycin, have also been used to secure remissions of the disease. Other medications employed are cytosine arabinoside, thioguanine and cyclophosphamide. An interesting drug for this condition, too, is L-asparaginase, an enzyme, which exerts its action by destroying the amino acid asparagine in the blood and extracellular fluids. Cancer cells must have asparagine to survive. All anti-cancer drugs are toxic and unpleasant reactions may occur from their use.

Attempts to use imunotherapy have also been tried. Live leukemic cells have been exchanged betwen leukemia patients. After an interval of time, the recipient's leukocytes were injected back into the donors. Definite improvement occurred in a series of young patients treated by this method.

Acute leukemia in adults is treated with the same drugs used in children. In adult chronic leukemias busulfan, 6-mercaptopurine, hydroxyurea, melphalan, thioguanine, chlorambucil, prednisone, cyclophosphamide and cytarabine are used. Radiation may also be employed.

HODGKIN'S DISEASE

Hodgkin's disease is a malignancy of lymphatic tissue and may be viral in origin. Usually, one group of lymph nodes enlarges and then others may follow. Fever is common and symptoms are determined by the pressure effects of the enlarging nodes. A strange symptom of the disease is that drinking of alcohol induces pain at one of the sites of involvement. When manifestations are well localized, intensive radiation will produce long remissions or even cures.

Advanced Hodgkin's disease is being treated with the drugs such as vincristine and prednisone, procarbazine, cyclophosphamide, BCNU, chlorambucil, or nitrogen mustard. Intensive intermittent use of several drugs has proven to be more effective than single drugs alone.

LUNG CANCER

Primary cancer of the lung has been constantly increasing for the last several decades. The usual sites of early involvement are in the bronchial tubes with later spread to the lungs. Only about 15% of these cancers are diagnosed when early and localized. Less than a third of lung cancers can be helped by surgery.

Diagnosis is made by x-ray examination, bronchoscopic examination with an electrically lighted instrument, biopsy of the tumor, and microscopic examination of the sputum or pleurisy fluids which may be present in the chest. Symptoms may be entirely absent early in the disease. When the patient finally comes to the physician he may complain of loss of appetite and weight, cough, raising of blood, associated infection and pain in the chest.

Implicated in the causation of primary lung cancer are coal tar fumes, oil sprays, benzol, chromates, arsenic, asbestos, iron oxide, nickel, nitrosamines, radioactive ores, hydrocarbons such as benzopyrene from industrial sources and automobile exhausts, air pollution and incinerator exhausts.

Cigarette smoking, in contrast to nonsmoking, is closely associated with cancer of the mouth, larynx, esophagus, lung, stomach, kidney, bladder, prostate and pancreas. The high ratio of lung cancer in cigarette smokers has convinced many physicians that the disease can be prevented by getting people to give up or never start smoking.

If lung cancer is detected early and localized, surgery may produce a permanent cure. Otherwise it is palliative only.

Useful drugs in treating lung cancer are nitrogen mustard, mechlorethamine, methotrexate, fluorouracil, chlorambucil, vincristine, cyclophosphamide, triethylenemelamine and its relative hexamethylmelamine. Radiation is employed in treating lung cancer and is often combined with surgery, occasionally with drug therapy. The salvage rate of lung cancer cases still leaves much to be desired. Prevention is still the best way to avoid dying of primary lung cancer. Quitting smoking and reducing exposure to occupational and environmental carcinogens may accomplish this purpose.

BREAST CANCER

Breast cancer occurs more frequently among unmarried women and childless married women. Breast cancer is rare among Japanese women, common in western women. Thyroid function is higher in the Japanese. Whether this plays a role in the disease incidence is unknown.

The first sign of breast cancer may be a lump in the breast, a mass or swelling in the axilla or armpit, inflammation of the breast which does not subside, or eczema of the nipple.

Small lesions should be excised. If large, a piece is removed (biopsy) for examination to determine whether it is cancer. Surgery has been an accepted method of treatment for breast cancer for many years. Either just the breast is removed, or the breast plus the adjacent muscles and lymph nodes in what is known as a radical resection. Sometimes radiation is used alone, when surgery is not possible, although it is often combined with surgery or used for recurrences of the cancer.

Castration, by surgical removal of the ovaries has been tried. If performed before the menopause, or within 1 year after menopause, about 40% of patients secure remission. Male hormones are often given to young women with breast cancer after removal of the ovaries, and female hormones are administered to women past the menopause or change of life. There is frequently a favorable remission. If both hormones fail, corticosteroids may be prescribed solely for the purpose of making the patient feel more comfortable.

Surgical removal of the adrenals or the pituitary gland may secure a good remission in about 50% of cases which previously had been surgically castrated and responded well.

Drugs may be tried when no more radiation can be given and the patient does not respond to hormone therapy. Nitrogen mustard will effectively reduce cancerous pleural fluid in the chest. Whether drug therapy along with surgery and/or radiation would enhance the attack on breast cancer is yet to be fully determined. Again, speculation arises as to the possibility of more powerful anticancer drugs being discovered, along with immunity procedures, to cure the disease. At the present time, the drugs used to treat breast cancer are cyclophosphamide, fluorouracil, thiotepa, methotrexate with or without vincristine, chlorambucil, male and female hormones and the corticosteroid prednisone.

UTERINE CANCER

Uterine cancer is more prevalent in married women than in nuns or single women, while the reverse is true in breast cancer. This fact, plus the correlation between early marriage and uterine cancer, suggests that sexual intercourse is an important provocateur in causing this malady.

It has been known for a long time that Jewish women, whose husbands are circumcised, have a very low incidence of cervical (neck of the womb) uterine cancer. The suspected carcinogen was believed to be the smegma under the male's foreskin. Later investigations indicated that promiscuous women had a higher incidence of uterine cancer. It was concluded that it was not the smegma per se that caused the disease, but something else was being transmitted. Studies have shown this agent to be a virus living in some smegmas. It is a type 2 herpes virus, which is related to the virus of "cold sores" and "shingles." Women with uterine cancer show a high antibody titre in their serums to this organism.

It should not be misconstrued by the reader that only promiscuous women have cervical uterine cancer. But if a woman is promiscuous, then her chances of being infected with type 2 herpes virus, constantly increases. It is possible for a virtuous woman to marry a man with this genital virus.

There may be no symptoms very early in uterine cancer, or the disease may be picked up on a routine examination with a Pap stain. As the malignancy advances there is a vaginal discharge, usually bloody. There may be pelvic discomfort or pain late in the course of the disease.

Cancer of the cervix of the uterus usually occurs in young women, and cancer of the body of the uterus is found more often in older women. Surgery very often will cure localized cancer in either of these areas. Radium is also very effective when placed in the cervix and/or body of the uterus. X-ray may be used in conjunction with radium where there is extension beyond the uterus.

Drugs used in treating uterine cancer are progestins, fluorouracil, cyclophosphamide, thiotepa and vincristine. However, they are not of striking value. Surgery and radiation of the womb produce a high rate of remissions.

PROSTATIC CANCER

Prostatic cancer is very common in males and it customarily occurs beyond the age of 45. Early diagnosis is often made on a routine rectal examination, when a small hard nodule can be found in the gland. Removal of the prostate at this time usually results in a cure.

There are no early symptoms. As the tumor enlarges, signs of obstruction appear. The patient has difficulty in urination and there may be bleeding in the urinary tract. Pain, weakness and loss of appetite occur. The malignancy often metastasizes to bone, and the first symptoms may be bone pain.

Surgery is resorted to initially to remove the growth. If there is extension beyond the prostatic region into bones or other areas, then castration is recommended, followed by female hormone therapy usually given as stilbestrol. Remissions are frequently attained by this treatment.

If stilbestrol is ineffective then other estrogenic and progesterone agents should be tried. Stilphosterol, medroprogesterone acetate and cyproterone acetate frequently produce remission when stilbestrol fails. In inoperable cases x-ray therapy is employed. Radiation effectively reduces prostatic size, stops bleeding and relieves bone pain. Radioactive phosphorus, intravenously, is also helpful in providing relief.

GASTROINTESTINAL CANCER

Stomach cancer is more prevalent in the Scandinavian countries, Iceland and Japan than in the USA. For some unknown reason, the incidence of stomach cancer has been declining in America for the last 25 years. In regions where stomach cancer is very common, people are on a high starch diet and consume very little fresh fruit and vegetables. In addition, they ingest smoked products and fermented foods which contain mycotoxins from bacteria or fungi. Liver cancer is rare in the USA, but common in parts of Africa and Asia where mycotoxins contaminate food.

Cancer of the colon shows no relationship, in world wide studies, to any diets or industrial diseases. However, it seems to be closely associated with ulcerative colitis and polyps of the colon, frequently developing when these disorders are present.

Burkitt, who discovered a herpes virus tumor in Africa which is now called Burkitt's tumor, indicates that there may be some connection between diet and rectal and colonic cancer. He notes that Americans ingest a highly refined diet which produces a concentrated and low residue. Consequently, this food gives rise to slow moving bowels, small hard feces and a lot of flatus (gas). Burkitt believes that this situation may contribute to appendicitis, diverticulitis, polyps, ulcerative colitis and cancer.

In contrast, Africans consume a bulky, unrefined, high residue diet and they have few of these diseases. American negroes and second generation Japanese on American refined diets, have more of these maladies than the natives in their former homelands.

Colon and rectal cancers are the most common malignancies of the gastrointestinal tract. Seventy five percent of these cancers arise in the anal, rectal, or sigmoid colon. Rectal finger examination will discover about one third of these tumors. As is true of most cancers, very early there are no symptoms. Signs leading to a suspicion of colon cancer are changes in bowel habits, bleeding from the rectum, abdominal pain, loss of appetite and weight, vomiting. Rectal cancer also is characterized by a change in bowel habits, rectal bleeding, weight loss, mucus in the stools and pain.

Surgery is the main treatment available. Drugs used to combat these cancers are fluorouracil and hydoxyurea.

SKIN CANCERS

Skin cancers are probably the most prevalent of all malignancies. The incidence of these growths is higher in the white race than in the black, because of the better pigment protection in negroes against sunlight. Redheads and natural blondes are more susceptible than olive complected individuals, for they have less pigment to sunscreen them.

Because early cancer of the skin is visible, in contrast to internal malignancies, it can be diagnosed and treated much quicker. It does not spread to distant areas as quickly as internal growths, so the opportunity for cure is much better. Sunlight appears to be the main inciting agent and ultraviolet radiation in animals will produce skin cancer. Areas of the skin exposed to the sun are the most frequent sites to develop cancer.

A skin growth that will not heal or that continues to grow, should be seen by a dermatologist or surgeon. If neglected the growth will probably ulcerate, bleed and become destructive to underlying tissue.

Treatment consists of surgical removal or electrosurgery with curetting. These methods yield a high percentage of cures. Radiation is reserved for poor surgical risks. Drugs are not used as a prime modality in treating skin cancer. Fluorouracil, bleomycin, TEIB, and DNCB, are being used along with a few other experimental drugs. The last two drugs are immunotherapeutic agents.

The most malignant of skin cancers is the malignant melanoma. Wide surgical excision is the recommended treatment. Drugs used for treating metastases are methotrexate, floxuridine and imidazole carboxamide. Immunotherapy has produced some remissions. The injection of BCG (the tuberculosis vaccine) directly into a melanoma nodule has also produced remission.

During the last 25 years a new specialty, oncology, devoted to studying tumorous growths has arisen. Surgery and radiation have been the prime methods for treating cancer, but have fallen far short of the goal of cure. Newer procedures have been coming into vogue such as hormonal, chemical, and immunological. Important advances are being made for controlling malignancies so as to prolong human life in comfort. Complete eradication and cure of cancer is coming closer to possibility. One day they will be here. Just when is still unknown.

Chapter Eighteen

DRUG INTERACTIONS

THE HUMAN BODY is a very complex biochemical machine. It is extremely versatile, and can ordinarily cope with new chemical molecules and compounds coming into its milieu. But at times these substances may be more than the body can handle, resulting in disruption, disorganization, and even death.

One condition that is encountered with medications is adverse reactions. While a drug is given for one purpose, an unwanted response may follow, and even a life threatening situation. Among the most common adverse reactions seen on an outpatient basis, according to Visconti and Smith, are those connected with oral contraceptives, antibiotics, corticosteroids, diuretics, hormones excluding oral contraceptives, tranquilizers and antidepressants. Contraceptives and antibiotics account for 40% of the reactions seen in these patients. The adverse reactions produced by these six classes of drugs have been described previously.

A distinction must also be made between drug incompatability and drug interaction. Incompatability may be noted in an intravenous bottle where two drugs have been inserted and a cloudy precipitate forms. However, incompataibility may occur in the bottle when there is no visible interaction, but where drugs inactivate themselves as in the case of the antibiotics kanamycin and methicillin (penicillin derivative). Penicillin-G is made impotent by phenylephrine because of its preservative bisulphite. Tetracycline antibiotics are photooxidized by riboflavin of the vitamin B complex. Levarterenol, blood pressure raiser for shock, will oxidize and become useless, unless dextrose sugar is mixed with the solution.

Drug interactions are variously defined. Hartshorn says they are phenomena which take place when the effects of one drug are modified by the previous or concomitant administration of the same or another drug. Stuart says drug interactions include reactions between various drugs, drugs and food, and drugs and disorders. All reactions may not be adverse, some may actually be beneficial.

We have observed that drugs may be modified or inactivated in an intravenous bottle. They may also deteriorate while lying on shelves, with liquids going faster than tablets or capsules. Therefore all these preparations have to be stamped with their expiration dates. Out of date drugs may be inert, harmless, or toxic. Drugs lying about and exposed to high temperatures may undergo chemical decomposition, becoming inert or toxic.

We have just seen that many things can happen to drugs before they ever get into the body. Equally important is what happens after medicines are given. Some drugs are more effective when injected than taken orally. In fact, medications like adrenalin and insulin are absolutely ineffective by the oral route. The gastrointestinal tract is an intricate chemical factory existing for the sole purpose of absorbing liquids and digested food products to keep the body alive. It contains acids, bases, complex proteins, enzymes, absorbent membranes, and other structures necessary for its functions. Drugs must come in contact with the various components of this system just like the foods and liquids.

Some drugs become inactivated in the gastrointestinal tract. Certain amines form insoluble complexes with the mucous proteins of the stomach and bowel. The tetracycline antibiotics form insoluble compounds with ions of aluminum, magnesium, calcium, bismuth and barium. To overcome this situation, agents such as citric acid, phosphates, and glucosamine are added to the tetracyclines to sort of restrain these ions and allow the complete absorption of the medication. Milk contains calcium and should not be given with tetracycline. Neither should drugs containing aluminum.

Enzymes in the gastrointestinal tract break down foods into digestable units. If a drug has similar chemical configurations to foods, it will also be digested and, instead of the medication entering the blood as such, a metabolic product either active or inactive will be absorbed. Drugs given by injection are more effective, and therefore smaller amounts are used. For there is no loss by digestive breakdown, intestinal inactivation, or poor obsorption.

Digestive processes may also be responsible for the toxicity of some drugs. Chloromycetin is much less injurious to the bone marrow when given by injection as opposed to oral administration. Holt believes this may be due to the formation of a toxic metabolic product, or possibly the drug interferes with some enzyme system. These interferences are strengthened by the fact that if the amino acid phenylalanine is given to man, or riboflavin of the vitamin B complex to animals, along with Chlormycetin, the toxicity to the bone marrow is reduced. Similarly, if large doses of vitamin B_6 and B_{12} are given children with cystic fibrosis, the optic neuritis caused by Chloromycetin can be reduced.

Some investigators claim that penicillin may not be the culprit responsible for penicillin drug allergy. The reaction they say, is probably due to a small amount of protein being attached to the drug and not removed in purification. When given intravenously or subcutaneously, the foreign protein may incite a severe allergic reaction. When the drug is given orally the protein may be digested off before absorption in the intestinal tract, thus lessening the chances of a fatal allergic response. This may or may not be the complete story of penicillin allergy.

While some drugs are affected by digestive enzymes, others are influenced by either the acid or lack of acid in the stomach. Some penicillins and the antibiotic erythromycin are inactivated by stomach acid, especially during the high acidity occurring when food is being digested in the organ. To circumvent this undesired reaction, acid sensitive drugs may be placed in a special coated material which will only dissolve in the gut. The medication can also be given between meals when stomach acid is low. A chemical derivative may be designed which will be resistant to the acid, or the drug can simply be given by injection.

Another factor becomes important in drug administration, and that is whether the drug is acid or alkaline. Acid type medications are absorbed from the stomach, while alkaline ones are assimilated from the intestine which is alkaline or neutral. Neutral drugs should be absorbed from either, but it is believed they are mostly absorbed from the intestine. Antacid medications would make the stomach more alkaline and hinder absorption of acid drugs, while substances that would make the intestines more acid would hinder absorption of alkaline medications.

Nonionized substances pass through cellular membranes more easily and are therefore more absorbable than substances which ionize and have electrical charges on them. For the membranes are made up of fatty-protein elements which have positive and negative charged groups. The charged ionic drugs are repelled by these membranes, while the un-charged nonionized drugs go through.

Another chemical principle that must be considered in administering drugs is solubility. Drugs are assimilated maximally when given in their salt form because they are more soluble. Many long acting drugs are incorporated into insoluble waxes, from which they gradually break out over a period of time and then become soluble and absorbed. Prolonged effects are also attained by suspending injectable drugs in oil or some other preparation such as silicone or beeswax.

The passage of drugs from the gut to the blood stream may be altered by other drugs. For example, the antibiotic neomycin prevents the absorption of penicillin, while the antibiotic puromycin stops the absorption of cholesterol. Allopurinol, the anti-gout medication, blocks the enzymes which limit the absorption of iron, causing an excessive assimilation of iron with toxic overtones.

Most drugs are insoluble in the blood. So they become bound to the albumin and globulin blood proteins, and this resulting complex is soluble. One drug may displace another drug from the protein-drug complex. The reason is not too clear. A more acid drug may pry loose a less acid one. It is known that the more acid preparations such as aspirin, the diuretic ethacrynic acid, the cholesterol lowering agent clofibrate, and the urinary-antiseptic nalidixic acid, displace quite easily the anticoagulants, thyroid hormones, oral antidiabetics, penicillin, and the antirheumatoid Butazolidine®.

In the blood, most drugs are protein bound, but a small portion exists free in a sort of equilibrium between the two states. When the free drug moves from the blood into the tissues, more of the bound drug becomes free. As the tissues metabolize the drug and excrete it, more moves in from the blood until all the medication is gone.

If a second drug enters the blood stream, while the first drug is still present, and displaces it, then a greater amount of the first preparation will be free to enter the tissues. This could well be a large overdose with serious consequences for the individual. In the case of anticoagulants this is especially true, for dosage is critical and too much of the medication will produce generalized bleeding and possibly a fatal hemorrhage.

The same principle holds true for other drugs. The anticancer drug methotrexate is administered in critical doses to treat malignancies. It has liver damaging potential. When excessive doses are set free in the body, serious and fatal results may follow. If oral antidiabetic drugs are detached from their bound form in too great a quantity, blood sugar will fall to very low levels. It has also been demonstrated by Solomon and his associates that foods, such as fatty acids, will displace some drugs from their protein attachments. In the case of sulfonamides, drug spinoff from the proteins is beneficial, for more of the drug will penetrate the tissues to strike down the bacteria.

In studying this phenomenon, Brodie suggests that the antirheumatic action of certain medications may be actually due to their detaching corticosteroids from their protein bindings. These steroids then produce the effect rather than their displacing agents.

Other drugs which act in this fashion are the muscle-paralyzer curare, certain antidepressants, and the antispasmodic atropine. The tranquilizer reserpine and some synthetic stimulating agents knock adrenalin and noradrenalin out of certain important sites in tissues. This action leaves a void for a period of time during which surgery would be hazardous, for these hormones maintain blood pressure.

In drug allergies, as for example penicillin, soluble complexes form between the drug and allergic antibodies. They may stay bound for months in the blood, with some free drug being released from time to time and showing up in allergic responses such as hives. This protein-allergen combination is eliminated very slowly, in some cases. When it breaks down temporarily, the complexes reform again, thus causing the long delay in recovering from the allergy.

Drugs leaving the blood, bind themselves to tissue proteins. Some tissues have a greater affinity for a particular medication than others. If a drug is bound at a site at which it is not directed, it may be loosened from this site and go to an active site if released by another drug or some body response.

An interesting drug is Antabuse®, given to alcoholics to prevent them from drinking. The medication inhibits an enzyme from metabolizing alcohol in the normal fashion and leaves it at the acetaldehyde stage. The accumulation of this substance in the body makes the alcoholic very sick. If he takes antabuse whenever he feels the urge to drink, the resulting discomfort may force him to quit drinking. It has been found that patients who are on Dilantin®, the anticonvulsive drug for epilepsy, when given Antabuse®, develop very high levels of Dilantin® in their blood with adverse reactions.

Drugs are metabolized in tissues, but the body's active factory for this is the omnipotent liver. Here, as in the tissues, two or more drugs may compete for the available metabolic enzymes, and the most active one is destroyed unwittingly, allowing the survivor to exert its action longer.

Until 1950 little was known about how drugs were metabolized by the body's enzymes. Brodie and his associates at the NIH found that the enzyme system of the liver was the main source for disposing of drugs. These potent synthesizers convert drugs from a fat solubility to a water solubility for the kidneys to excrete.

It was observed a few years ago that drugs like phenobarbital, the sedative chloral hydrate, or the antihistamines, stimulated the liver's enzyme system. If a second drug was then administered, it would be metabolized much quicker, especially if it was another barbiturate or an anticoagulant which prevents blood clotting. The amount of increase was about 10 to 20 times the ordinary rate. Researchers have now identified over 200 substances that increase enzyme production in the liver. This includes halogenated insecticides, food additives, carcinogenic chemicals and even nicotine.

This fact has important significance. For if a patient is taking both phenobarbital and the anticoagulant Coumadin® larger doses of the latter are needed. If suddenly the phenobarbital is stopped, the inactivation of the anticoagulant ceases. There is now a build-up of the latter drug, which actually reaches an overdose stage. The patient starts to bleed, and, if the condition is not quickly corrected, the patient may hemorrhage to death. Similar interactions have occurred between the anticoagulants and chloral hydrate, antihistamines, antiepileptic drugs, various sedatives, and the insecticide chlordane.

Even carcinogenic benzpyrene, found in cigarette smoke, stimulates the enzyme system. Some investigators believe that lung cancer may only develop in individuals who are unable to respond with an increased metabolic effect to destroy or inactivate the benzpyrene.

Liver enzymes inactivate the anti-gout drug allopurinol, the stimulant Ritalin®, the female estrogenic hormones, the antifungus drug griseofulvin, some antibiotics, and orally taken antidiabetic preparations. If another medication is taken at the same time as one of these drugs, and it effects the enzyme system too, its action may be drastically altered.

In the chapter on Psychic Drugs it was pointed out that the monoamine oxidase enzyme system is inhibited by antidepressant drugs such as Parnate®, Mardil®, and the blood-pressure-lowering agent Eutonyl®. As a result, this system can no longer neutralize stimulating drugs like amphetamines, ephedrine, guanethidine, and tyramine which may be ingested by consuming wines, cheeses, and pickled herring. Certain drugs bought by people in drug stores without prescriptions may contain activators. This is especially true of cold medicines (containing ephedrine, phenylephrine, and phenylpropanolamine). These stimulating drugs when taken by individuals, who are already taking the antidepressant drugs mentioned above, may create a serious high-blood-pressure crisis with fatal results.

It will be obvious from the above, and other discussions in this chapter, that patients should not be taking medications without their physician's knowledge. For such medications may effect the action of prescription drugs. Smoking, alcohol, hallucinogenic and psychogenic drugs, and environmental pollutants may all be involved in drug interactions.

An interesting observation by Bockner and Roman is that contraceptive drugs produce increased binding of substances such as iron, the thyroid-hormone thyroxine, and the lipid (fat) fraction of the blood. This phenomenon results from an increased production of blood proteins. The surplus proteins binds more substances. This effect may explain why the fatty triglycerides rise in the blood and the drug clofibrate loses its ability to lower cholesterol.

Whether this is a factor in producing blood clots in the veins of women using contraceptives is not clear at present.

Strange are the ways of metabolism. Some people convert the sweetening agent cyclamate into the suspected carcinogenic-chemical called cyclohexylamine. Williams of St. Mary's Hospital in London found the reason why. The bacterial metabolism in their intestines produced this substance, for absorption into the blood not the individual's own body metabolism.

Also intriguing is the story of certain liver-damaging drugs such as carbon tetrachloride and bromobenzene. It was believed that these chemicals harm the liver as soon as they enter it. But Brodie showed that an enzyme system in the liver of rats oxidizes these substances into very unstable and toxic chemicals. But they remain stable just long enough to destroy the liver cells and possibly the host too.

Interesting, too, is the discovery of Riegelman and associates who found that phenobarbital increases bile secretion from the liver. This action accelerates the passage of the antifungus drug griseofulvin through the gastrointestinal tract, and thus reduces the amount absorbed.

A bizarre finding is that blood groupings may play a role in disease. People with blood group O are not as likely to develop clots in their veins as those with groups A and B. Women with type O blood taking contraceptives, can expect less clotting in their veins than type A or B. This virtue turns into a liability in ulcer patients, for type O is more likely to have hemorrhages than A or B.

Patients with low albumin-protein levels in their blood and taking the corticosteroid prednisone have adverse reactions. The reason is that there is not enough albumin in the blood to bind the drug, and so there is too much free prednisone to react with tissues. Individuals with normal albumin levels do not have this difficulty.

The excretion of drugs provides additional interactions. Most drugs which are not metabolized are excreted chiefly in the urine, although an occasional drug is eliminated in the milk, lungs, or bile.

Free circulating drugs in the blood are mostly fat soluble. As they circulate through the filtering apparatus of the kidney they are reabsorbed back into the circulation if they have not become ionized. If the urine is markedly acid or alkaline, the drugs acquire ionization charges and are then excreted. Weak acids like aspirin, Butazolidine®, and phenobarbital are more rapidly excreted in an alkaline urine. This knowledge is of advantage when patients have an overdose of such drugs. A weak base like amphetamine is more rapidly excreted in an acid urine. Devotees of "speed" who know this, prolong the effect of the drug by taking the alkalizer bicarbonate.

Therefore, when prescribing medications, it becomes important to know whether other drugs are being given and if they are producing an acid or alkaline urine. Drugs causing an alkaline urine are sodium bicarbonate, sodium carbonate, mercurial diuretics, and the diuretics Daimox® and Cardrase®. Acidifying drugs are ammonium chloride, glutamic acid hydrochloride, and sodium acid phosphate.

The urinary antiseptics, mandelic acid and methenamine, are only effective in acid urine. Methenamine is broken down to the antiseptic formaldehyde in acid urine. Some sulfa drugs may precipitate out in acid urine, blocking the kidneys. That is why sodium bicarbonate is prescribed with these drugs.

The kidney has a secretory mechanism also for eliminating drugs, presumably by some kind of enzyme action. Drugs eliminated by this method are penicillin, salicyclic acid, certain diuretics, the antiinflammatory agent indomethacin, and the antigout medication probenecid. If penicillin and probenecid are given at the same time, however, the secretion of penicillin is blocked and penicillin levels will remain up in the blood. Probenecid will do the same for the diuretic ethacrynic acid, and may also potentiate the action of the oral antidiabetic drugs.

This phenomenon of inhibition of kidney excretion is also noted when small doses of salicylates, ethacrynic acid, the antituberculosis drug Pyrazinamide® and the diuretic Chrorthalidone® block the secretory mechanism and cause the uric acid levels to rise in the blood. Larger doses of salicylates plus probenecid inhibit the reabsorption of uric acid and causes increased elimination. Strangely, too, salicylates may interfere with the uric acid lowering effects of probenecid, the antirheumatic Butazolidin®, and the cholesterol lowering clofibrate.

Some drugs produce additional effects to those for which they are mainly employed. Antibiotics such as polymycin, neomycin, streptomycin, kanamycin, and several others induce muscle relaxation. This action is intensified when kidney excretion is slow or ulcers in the gastrointestinal tract allow increased absorption of these drugs. One should be very cautious about using these agents if muscle relaxers such as curare, succinyl choline or similar agents are being administered. Neostigmine antagonizes the action of neomycin, kanamycin, and streptomycin, but has no effect on the others.

When a person is on barbituates or tranquilizers and drinks alcohol, the interaction increases the effect of these drugs. Deaths may occur and have frequently followed alcohol-barbiturate indulgence. Alcohol enhances the central nervous system depression of antihistamines and tricyclic antidepressants.

When an individual is on analgesics, anticoagulants, antihistamines, antiepileptics, steroids, hypnotics, and on the antifungus griseofulvin, the ingestion of phenobarbital inhibits all these drugs. Phenobarbital also enhances the metabolism of male and female hormones.

The tetracycline antibiotics are inhibited by antacids. In turn, they inhibit penicillin if it is given simultaneously. Penicillin is inhibited by antacids and Chloromycetin®. The sulfa drugs are inhibited by antacids, potentiated by probenecid, enhance the action of oral antidiabetics and the anticancer drug Methotrexate®.

The anticoagulant Dicumarol® is inhibited by antacids and the sedative chloral hydrate. The anticoagulant Coumadin's® action is increased by salicylates, thyroxine hormone, the antiepileptic Dilantin®, and the hormone Nilevar®.

The activity of the oral antidiabetics is enhanced by the anticoagulant coumarin, the diuretic ethacrynic acid, insulin, and thyroxine.

Most blood pressure lowering agents are inhibited by amphetamines, while the thiazides usually enhance the action.

We have observed, in general, the many variables that may occur between the time a drug is prepared for use and its eventual action, metabolic fate, possible inhibition and antagonism, and finally its excretion. There are also genetic differences in people that may alter their ability to cope with drugs. Sjoqvist of Sweden and Gillette of the NIH found that patients taking medications for chronic diseases did not always maintain constant blood drug-levels despite the fact that they were on the same drug dosage. Some had very high levels and developed side effects while others had low levels and received no therapeutic results from the medications. These marked differences indicate genetic variables.

It has been found, too, that the administration of a standard dosage of certain drugs, such as the antituberculosis-drug isoniazid, to normal subjects disclosed that some were fast inactivators and had low blood levels, while others were slow inactivators and had high blood levels. The fast inactivators possessed an acetylating enzyme lacking in the slow inactivators. There is a low incidence of slow inactivation among Eskimos and Orientals, while a higher incidence up to 50% is present in Whites and Negroes. Slow inactivators are the only ones that get a toxic nerve reaction with the drug. The response of tuberculosis patients to the drugs is not influenced by their genetic type.

LaDue of New York University noted genetic differences in a random study of patients taking the same drugs. Identical twins, presumably possessing the same genetic makeup, excreted various drugs at the same rate. Fraternal twins, presumably not having an identical genetic makeup, excrete the same drugs at different rates.

Individual variations may be serious when there are hereditary abnormalities. One of the best known of these is the deficiency of the enzyme known as glucose-6-phosphate dehydrogenase, a chemical reducing enzyme which maintains the integrity of the red blood cells. When drugs are given, with oxidizing properties to such patients, the red blood cells are destroyed (hemolytic anemia). Among these medications are phenacetin, acetanilid, sulfonamides, the antimalarial primaquine, and others. This trait is present in up to 14% of American Negroes, 10% of Greeks, and up to 35% in African and Mediterranean groups.

Another serious situation exists in patients unable to hydrolyze the drug succinylcholine, which paralyzes the voluntary muscles of respiration for deep relaxation during surgery. Instead of acting for only 5 minutes as in normals, the drug may paralyze respiration for many hours, calling for artificial respiration. Those who rapidly hydrolyze the drug may seem immune to its effects and require massive doses for therapy.

Special consideration must be given to drug usage and drug dosage in youngsters. Very young children absorb drugs differently than adults because their intestine is relatively underdeveloped and they have a more rapid transit through their gastrointestinal tract. Their enzymes systems and excretory mechanisms are still immature. Children have a higher water content than adults and a relatively greater body surface. Ignoring these special considerations may result in no therapeutic response or severe adverse drug reactions. One of the most striking examples of this is the "gray syndrome" caused by the failure of the immature liver to bind Chloromycetin® by a process known as conjugation and the inability of the kidneys to excrete the free drug circulating in the blood.

Mirkin, in summarizing drug data, showed that in newborn infants some drugs are more toxic and others less toxic than in adults. More toxic are phenobarbital, morphine, chloral hydrate, aspirin, the tranquilizer chlorpromazine, and the anticoagulant Dicumarol®. Less toxic are amphetamines, strychinine, digitalis, codeine, and Demerol®.

Special situations can occur in children. For example, oxygen in premature infants can be highly toxic and cause eye damage. Vitamin K, sulfa drugs, and others can produce a bile staining of the brain. Tetracyclines can give rise to dental staining of permanent teeth. Growth may be retarded by long continued use of the corticosteroids.

Body metabolism is a complex, integrated process. Most drugs introduced into this dynamic situation are foreign substances. Just what their fate will be, and what the ultimate effects are going to be on the living machine, is of ultimate concern both to the physician and the human recipient. There are both observable and unobservable events on the road to therapeutics.

Circumstances along the way such as genetic defects in digestion or metabolism, variable absorption phenomena, bacterial influences, acidity neutrality and alkalinity, dispersal in the circulation and tissues, enzymatic action, along with chemical and metabolic alterations, all play a role in the eventual fate of drug and man.

Chapter Nineteen

DRUGS AND THE BIOLOGICAL TIME CLOCK

It was once believed that in a healthy animal or person certain physiologic values were constant and immutable, and were only altered in disease. Drugs were given to shift the values present in disease back to normal. Therefore, with this concept, one only had to know the actions of drugs to prescribe them for various disorders. In the last 20 years, it has been evident that there are drug interactions, and knowledge of these phenomena is now necessary to successfully administer medications.

If this was the whole story, things would be relatively but not absolutely easy. However, it has been learned that the normal animal body is an intricate, integrated, physio-chemical entity which is in a dynamic state of unstable equilibrium. Billions of chemical reactions are going on at all times, which are impossible to comprehend by the finite human mind at a given moment, and they are not stabilized at a given level. Blood pressure, blood sugar, temperature and other characteristics of the human or animal body are constantly being altered, not set at an absolute value.

What is the cause of this unsteady state, why does it exist, how is it related to disease, and what is its purpose? Furthermore, how does it effect drugs that are administered and how do drugs effect it? This most intriguing phenomenon which we shall explore is known, for lack of a better term, as the Biological Time Clock.

Drugs, Demons, Doctors, and Disease

Stewart Wolf, in looking for a new cause for disease, first reviewed man's past quests. For thousands of years man blamed outside hostile forces as well as himself. Pasteur's work seemed to indicate that outside hostile agents, namely the bacteria, were the prime antagonists. At the same time another Frenchman by the name of Pidoux claimed that disease was the interplay of both external and internal factors.

The Chinese, thousands of years ago, believed in a dual system of controls (mentioned in Chapter 2 on Ancient Medicine). This was the Yin and Yang. The former is the cold, negative, female influence of the universe, while the latter is the warm, positive, male influence. The interplay of these opposing forces determines a man's health. If out of balance, disease occurs. When finely tuned, health predominates.

Stewart Wolf, in analyzing disease today, notes that in some cases of diabetes the patient, instead of having a scarcity of insulin, actually has a surplus. But antagonists and binding substances prevent the insulin from working. The pancreas, heeding the demand of the body for more insulin, pours it on, and something else reacts by producing more binders and antagonists, possibly antibodies to insulin. Similarly, in pernicious anemia, the intrinsic factor necessary to prevent anemia is present in adequate amounts but prevented from acting. Normally the body is in equilibrium between creating and eliminating red blood cells, but in hemolytic anemia the body is destroying them faster than it can make them.

It has become apparent that the systems which regulate the body are subject to definite cyclic rhythms. These "Biologic Moods," if we can call them such, are affected by cosmic stimulation and may occur on a yearly, seasonal, monthly, weekly, or daily basis.

In fact the whole universe performs in a definite cadence. There are still remnants of slow-radiation pulsations in the vast reaches of the universe, which date from the original Big Bang explosion when the universe was created billions of years ago. At that time, the gigantic holocaust hurled huge amounts of galactic matter outward into the cosmos, and these masses have been moving away from each other ever since at fantastic speeds. The galaxies rotate in rhythmic form as they move through space. The stars, planets, moons, and comets, as well as space debris, also rotate in definite patterns. Life, which is a microcosm of the universe, must therefore conform to rhythmic cycles.

Drugs, Demons, Doctors, and Disease

According to Mock and his associates, the body alternates between retaining and excreting salt and water. These cycles fluctuate every few days. Diuretics are effective when given at the peak of retention, but are ineffective when administered at the end of the cycle.

Wolf showed that motor movements of the stomach, in a fasting person, appear every 3 hours and last for 20 minutes. If a motor stimulating drug is given at the end of this period, it produces no response. Halberg discovered that the toxin of bowel bacteria (the colon bacilli) will kill 85% of mice when injected at noon, but only 5% of mice when injected at midnight. These observations indicate that drug effects are more potent at certain times and certainly less effectual or ineffective at others.

Damage to the brain may cause disease, as was first noted by the appearance of sugar in the urine, by Claude Bernard in the last century. Harvey Cushing in this century demonstrated the production of peptic ulcers by brain lesions. Gunn produced irregular heart rhythms and even caused the blood's cholesterol to rise after stimulation of the brain. These experiments indicate that interfering with the regulating control of the brain will induce tissue damage.

Strangely, too, an overactive defensive mechanism may cause disease. This is true in the disease known as lupus erythematosus. If the defensive mechanism is blunted by the corticosteriods, the patient may improve and his life be prolonged. Rowe and his co-workers demonstrated that if rats received x-ray and then were injected by a nerve damaging virus, nothing happened. But rats not radiated and receiving the same virus all died. In the radiated group the virus could be recovered in the body, but no disease developed. This was due to the radiation destroying the capacity of the white cells to attack the virus, and, if this is not done, manifestation of the disease will appear.

Stress may also cause disease. Monkeys in a zoo, harboring disease producing parasites and apparently quite well, will get sick when moved to a new environment. Wolf suggests that new types of stress may be responsible for the frequent recurrences of cold sore infections (herpes virus) in humans.

Hans Selye has shown by many experiments that constant or frequent stress will produce the General Alarm Syndrome. In this state the body's defenses adapt quickly, but then lose their ability to cope with continued tension. As they become exhausted, various tissues in the body degenerate. If the situation is not terminated the animal will die.

Stewart Wolf, in analyzing his data, believes that health or disease is the product of the rhythmic interaction of stimulating and inhibitory powers in the body, just like the old Chinese concept of Yin and Yang. Wide swings of the cycles may cause disease, while a proper equilibrium will insure health through the regulatory centers of the brain.

Additional investigators reveal rhythmic cycles in insects. Cole and Adkinson studied the most effective way to kill boll weavils with parathion. They found that a dose used at dawn killed 10% of the insects and a similar dose used 3 hours later eradicated 90%. This illustrated the effect of light and a photoperiodic rhythm. Other researchers working with the housefly and cockroaches noted that they were especially vulnerable to insecticides about 4 P.M.

Franz Halbert, of the University of Minnesota Medical School, has extensively studied biologic rhythms. He kept mice in a stable environment of 12 hours of light and 12 hours of darkness. He discovered that certain white cells known as eosinophiles (because they have a speckled red appearance when stained with the red dye eosin) are highest in mouse blood during the middle hours of light and fall to practically nothing during the middle of darkness. The cortisol level of the blood is rising while the eosinophile cells are dropping. Such peaks and valleys of definite recurring periods every 24 hours Halberg called "circadian" (from the Latin "circa" meaning about and "dies" meaning daily).

Halberg and associates demonstrated that this light synchronized cycling was present in many tissues, organs, and systems of the body. Various phenomena related to it are blood sugar, temperature, the cellular growth and metabolism of various tissues such as skin, hair, adrenals, pancreas, and liver. Presumably all living things have circadian periodicity as well as other biological clocks.

Lawrence Scheving of the Chicago Medical School explored the relationship of administered drugs to circadian rhythms in rats. He found that if he gave deadly doses of amphetamines at certain hours, up to 78% of the rodents expired. At other times as few as 6% perished. Similar results were seen with nicotine, strychinine, pentobarbital (nembutal), and other drugs. Scheving concluded from his experiments that man, like the rat, is a composite of many physiological rhythms, and that variations in resistance depend upon the changing phases of these cycles.

Reinberg of the National Scientific Research Center of Paris emphasizes the fact that there are altered responses to drugs, such as histamin, and also to allergy skin testing at various times of the day or night. All this suggests to him that we should reevaluate eventually the study of drugs, toxicity, and therapeutics on a biologic time clock basis.

An interesting comparison is made between man and mouse. The rodent is a night wandering animal and therefore produces most of his cortisol during the daytime hours. Man, who is a daytime primate, builds up his cortisol during the night. But he excretes most of his in the early hours of the morning, with gradually diminishing amounts being cast out during the rest of the day. Ideally then, adrenal steroid drugs should be given during the morning.

Man's circadian rhythms become important, it has been learned, when he jet travels to the East or West. North and South travel creates no problems for we are in the same time zone. When four or more time zones are quickly passed through, in an easterly or westerly direction, our biologic time clocks are disturbed. We can make up our sleep loss quickly, but it takes about a week for our biologic rhythms to be reset to the new time zone, with the east to west zone readjusting more quickly. During this interval, because of the discordant arrythmia, a person is not at his peak efficiency for conferences, business transactions, or anything demanding keen perspicacity.

Interesting facts on human cyclical rhythms have been discovered. There is an alternating opening and closing of the nasal passages in most people. While one side closes down quite a bit, the other opens up wider. Control for this reaction is probably in the central nervous system. According to Hamilton and coworkers blood levels of iron decrease during the day when adrenal action is most evident, and increases during sleep when the adrenal action slows down. Killman and associates showed that bone marrow cells are increasingly active during the day reaching a peak at midnight then becoming sluggish.

The cycles of blood cells are periodic. Certain white cells known as neutrophiles, and they make up the majority of the white cells, are most numerous in the blood during the day. The red cells and monocytic white cells peak during the evening. The eosinophilic and lymphocytic white cells are highest at night.

Urinary output of water and electrolytes show a sharp increase around the forenoon with a marked peaking of potassium excretion at midday. This is considered an excellent reference cycle for evaluating circadian rhythms.

The human heart possesses a circadian rhythm, with minimum rates in the morning and maximum rates later in the day. Isolated heart cells growing in cultures develop a pulsating rhythm. As masses of these cells develop in the culture they assume a synchronous beat. The normal heart is an integrated mass of cells responding to an electric discharging mechanism (SA node) which is under nervous and hormonal control.

The SA node establishes normal rhythm by discharging impulses from the right upper (atrial) wall of the heart. In heart implants, the SA nodal area of the right atrium of the recipient's heart is left in, after the diseased heart is removed. The new donor heart, which has no nerve control, is sutured to this area. We now have two SA nodes. Kraft and his associates demonstrated two different rhythms, detectable on the electrocardiogram, in an implant case they studied. Each node maintained its own particular rhythm, but the donor heart followed only its own pacemaker. A circadian rhythm of 23.4 hours was established for both SA nodes. The donor heart's pacemaker, however, preceded the recipient pacemaker by 135 minutes in the 23.4 hour rhythmic cycle.

Like the heart, Berlyne and his group showed that a transplanted cadaver kidney (removed at the moment of death for transplanting) has a diurnal rhythm in its excretion of water and kidney wastes. However, there is a greater phase shift from the rhythm it had established before transplant surgery. This is about 12 hours or 180°, while the donor heart was out of phase by 2 hours or 30°

In trying to probe into the living cells to see how and where the rhythms start, Britton Chance of the Pennsylvania School of Medicine, studied yeast and beef heart cells. Chance observed oscillating processes in the cytoplasm (protoplasm of the cell) and also in the mitochondria (small metabolic granules in the cytoplasm). He feels these rhythmic pulsations are enzyme fired at cycles of 1 to 2 minutes, and calls them the busy balance wheels which tick off the earthly days and years of animal and plant life.

To describe this phenomenon Chance uses the term feedback enzyme oscillator. The mechanism consists of three steps, two of which are enzyme stroked. First there is a buildup, then an inhibition, then the rhythm starts again.

Circadian rhythms have been demonstrated in the nervous structure of lower organisms, even when the structure was separated from the rest of the body. Some researchers have conditioned single nerve cells to fire off impulses at regular intervals. The human brain gives off wave recordings which can be visualized on the electroencephalogram. Man's cyclic variations are no better than that of bees or plants, but only more complex. Researchers have observed that the regularity of stress-inducing stimulation in animals creates neuroses. Similarly, they reason, the arbitrary working habits imposed on men today may lead to physical and physiological disorders, especially in occupations with the daily monotony of assembly-line work.

According to biologist John Palmer of New York University, man designates time in seconds, hours, weeks, years, cocktail hours, and vacation times, all of which are artifacts of our present civilization. At present a day is 24 hours, but 370 million years ago it was 22 hours. The question that immediately occurs is, were the circadian rhythms of that period based on a 22 hour day? Frankly, we may never know.

The 24-hour cycle says Palmer, is universal for man, animals, and plants. If man is isolated from sunlight, either deep in a cave or in a soundproof laboratory with no daylight, man automatically adjusts to eating, sleeping, and activating around a 24-hour schedule. Animals subjected to similar laboratory conditions exhibit a continual circadian rhythmicity. The human infant does not have a sleep-wake rhythm established until about the third week.

Human body temperature is not really 98.6 degrees. It varies over a 24-hour period being lowest in the morning and rising to its highest point in the late afternoon. Man's mental acumen and physical performance peak between 1-7 P.M. and reach their lowest point between 2-6 A.M. Experiments show a close relationship between body temperature changes and efficiency. There are *morning people* who rise early, work, perform, and learn best in the morning hours. Their temperatures peak before noon. *Evening people* become maximum performers in late afternoon or early evening and their temperatures peak in similar manner. It becomes obvious that metabolic processes operate faster at higher temperatures.

Palmer points out that infrequent happenings are also rhythmic motivated. The rate of childbirth is highest between 2-7 A.M., and the death rate is also greatest during this same period. Women tend to begin menstruation most often during the wee hours of the morning.

Life, if it is to exist, must conform to cosmic influences. Because of the sun, living things have circadian rhythms. We also have a close neighboring planet which strongly effects our earth, and that is the moon. Once the moon was much closer to us scientists say, and tides were higher and stronger. Many marine animals living along the seashore today have adjusted to the 12 hour cyclical rise and fall of the seas caused by moon pull.

The time between new moons, or the synod-lunar month, is 29.5 days. There are many rhythms in lower marine animals with periods of 29.5 days. Aristotle knew that the egg production of the Mediterranean sea urchins was highest at the time of full moon and advised gourmets to collect these delicacies at this time for consumption.

The moon was believed at one time to cause insanity, hence the name lunacy. There have been few studies to confirm or deny this traditional thinking.

Menstruation, says Palmer, is actually a 29.5 day cycle instead of 28 days. This fits into the concept of lunar influence. The average gestation or pregnancy period is 266 days or 9 lunar months. In checking the birth dates of over one quarter million children born in New York City municipal hospitals, Palmer found the highest conception rate is during the three days around the full moon, suggesting an increased mating activity, also characteristic of lower animals.

The famous "Black Out Power Failure" of the East coast of the USA occurred on November 9, 1965. Just nine months later, the birthrate jumped in New York City hospitals. Newspapers said it was the complete darkness which stimulated the matings and the ecologists were wrong. The papers were wrong, for it was the night of the full moon.

There is also a rhythm in the human female's sexual desire. Libido was highest during the latter half of menstruation and during the period prior to ovulation.

One of the most important aspects of the ticking biologic time-clock is the response of humans or animals to various toxins and medications at different hours. If identical doses of bacterial toxins are injected into mice, 80% are killed at 8 P.M. while less than 20% succumb at midnight. Alcohol killed all mice when injected at 8 P.M. but only 20% of a sample population at 8 A.M. Sodium pentobarbital (Nembutal), given for anesthesia to rats, produced 66% longer unconsciousness at night than in identical daytime doses. Damage by x-ray is more extensive at night than during the day.

These reactions are probably due to variations in the cyclic rhythms of the enzymes of the liver and other tissues to detoxify these toxins and drugs. If they are out of phase with the toxic agents disorders, disease, or death will follow.

Allergic responses in many vary with the time of day. Skin testing for allergens shows the most reaction at 11 P.M. and the least reaction at 11 A.M. The same reaction occurs with histamine at these time periods. The night reaction represents the low point in circadian rhythm for the adrenal glands. This periodicity may account for the prevalence of asthmatic attacks at night. The bronchial tubes are more sensative to histamine during this time period. Allergic individuals are also more sensitive to their allergens during this period. Aspirin remains in the circulation a shorter length of time if taken at night than during the day.

Pertinent questions are bound to arise as the cyclical studies of man are advanced. Should heart beat rhythms match before transplantation, and should kidney phases be in harmony too? Should people be operated upon in the morning or at night if they are "evening" or "day" people? When is the best time to match the patient with his medication?

Paul Williamson emphasizes that every human action has a certain rhythmicity and this includes eating, sleeping, bowel elimination, dying, mental functions, and possibly obesity. The mind will not tolerate rhythmic deviations easily. Such reaction will be noted in a girl whose menstrual period suddenly becomes too early or too late. The sex act is rhythmic and, if off balance, there is a sharp response. For some there is rhythmic polygamy and, if blocked, the mind becomes intolerant.

The human brain has a cyclical pattern as observed on the electroencephalogram. It is conceivable that abnormal rhythms, not measurable at present, are the cause of schizophrenia and other psychic disorders, because the patient cannot tolerate them, according to Williamson. The human mind does not easily endure alterations in periodicity. The horrendous results of our civilization produce the frequent assaults on our rhythmicity. It is not surprising, therefore, that psychoneuroses are so common as to practically be the normalcy of our times. We use drugs to help these people to bear their arrythmicity, not to correct it.

According to Adel Ismail, male sexual desires are more intense in the morning for the male sexual hormones are highest in the blood between 4 A.M. and noon. He believes that women have a similar cycle with their female hormones. He laments the situation by pointing out that modern man rushes for the commuter train in the morning while his mate in robe and curlers, possibly passionate too, tackles the housework.

A. Louis Southren says that due to the rhythmic production of male sex hormone, there may be a best time for administering the hormone for various abnormalities. He states than men and women produce the same hormones, but normal men produce about 20 times more male hormone than do normal women. Some masculine types of women produce more male hormone than normal women. These women are said to be more susceptible to uterine cancer. There is a cyclic rise and fall in the blood levels of male hormone, but in women the level is pretty constant.

For years the function of the small pineal gland, situated very nearly in the center of the brain, was unknown. Axelrod of the NIH (National Institute of Health), and Wurthman of MIT have made some very exciting discoveries which help us to understand the contribution of the pineal gland to the body's ecology and its participation in biological rhythms.

These men found that light was the stimulant for the pineal tissue to spring into action. With the exception of birds, where light may penetrate through their heads, other animals receive light excitation from the eye's retina over brain pathways to the pineal gland. If this latter route is severed, the gland is not energized.

If activated, pineal noradrenalin changes pineal serotonin to melatonin. The latter hormone is so-called because it lightens the color of the skin by inhibiting the pigment cells (melanocytes) from producing skin pigment (melanin). Melatonin also influences the thyroid gland, sex glands, brain wave tracings, and induces sleep. Melatonin may function by direct action on the brain because injection of the hormone increases the quantity of serotonin in the brain. Pineal noradrenalin, pineal serotonin, and melatonin all have circadian rhythms. Pineal noradrenalin drives the pineal rhythms of the other two chemicals.

Serotonin is more widely distributed in the nervous system than melatonin. It is found, too, in the intestine, blood, animals, plant tissues, fruits, nuts, and insect venoms. Brain serotonin is believed to be involved in behavior and mood changes. The tranquilizer reserpine depletes the brain of serotonin and thereby winds down psychoses. Some think that serotonin is connected with schizophrenia. Drugs which block serotonin produce insomnia.

Brain noradrenalin rhythm is the reverse of the timing of pineal noradrenalin rhythm. The hypothalmic regions of the brain, quite close to the pineal organ, follow the brain noradrenalin cycling. The hypothalamus controls body and brain temperature, glandular activity, such as the adrenals, which all follow a circadian periodicity. Noradrenalin presumably drives these rhythms and is probably the instrument to stimulate nerve activity. It may be, therefore, the drummer boy that causes us to follow the beat of the changing daily rhythms, and it may be responsible for sleeping, waking, eating, digesting, agility, alertness, and other biologic needs necessary for adjusting to a capricious world.

Noradrenalin is formed from the amino acid tyrosine which is present in protein food. The levels of tyrosine and other amino acids rise and fall in the blood in a predictable fashion every 24 hours. Tyrosine is also utilized for making the skin pigment melanin, the thyroid hormone thyroxine, and adrenalin. It is also helpful in converting fats and proteins into energy-useful sugar. Amino acid fluctuation in the blood may be influenced by the adrenal hormones and insulin, not the protein diet.

The circadian rhythm of the amino acids in the blood may indicate the best time for biologic synthesis in the body. If the amount of these substances in the blood is critical, and certain of these protein building blocks such as tyrosine, tryptophan, and methionine, are usually present in small quantities, then there may be a limitation of material at times for the various organs, tissues, and brain to make their essential proteins.

Wurtman, Axelrod, and their associates believe that there must be a master timeclock in the nervous system which coordinates all the body's biological clocks with the outside world. Unifying these concepts with medicine and psychiatry should bring some exciting developments in the near future.

Certain questions come to mind in the opinion of these investigators. Will more understanding of the pineal organ tell us why certain nervous disorders become more severe during certain seasons? Why do ulcers flare in the spring and fall? Will manipulation of the pineal gland by light and darkness be of help in the treatment and prevention of disease? If so light may become a drug for useful purposes. Will it be used to augment drug therapy, and will drugs be given at the proper biologic time to be more potent in treatment? Will x-ray therapy and surgery be tuned to the timeclock of circadian rhythms instead of man's present chronologic clock? Will a person's job be equated with his cyclic rhythm for maximum performance?

Frank Brown of Northwestern University demonstrated that Long Island oysters, which presumably open and close their shells synchronously with the tides, developed a new rhythm when moved to Evanston, Illinois. This change was shown to be dependent upon the moon being positioned at zenith over the city. The oysters obviously were influenced by lunar position, not tides.

John Cottrell cites other curious lunar phenomena. The waning moon is a signal to adult eels to leave Europeon rivers and migrate 3,000 miles back to the warm Sargasso Sea where they were born. Tropical worms known as Palolos live in coral rock and emerge twice a year on the first day of October and November when the moon goes into its final quarter. The biggest hauls of herring occur at full moon. All these marine animals react the same way even if the moon is obscured by heavy clouds. Strangely, the oysters responded even when kept indoors where no moonlight could reach them. Cottrell raises the question as to why the moon should not influence humans, if it exerts an effect on living creatures as well as the vast seas.

The electromagnetism of the upper atmosphere changes with the phases of the moon. It definitely alters man's behavior. It is claimed that negative atmospheric ions are beneficial. Positive ions are harmful and aggravate sinus infections, asthma, rhinitis, and hay fever. They also induce headache, fatigue and dizziness. Negative ions relieve these disorders. The World Meteorological

Organization states that air ions produce physiological changes in bacteria, fungi, plants, and mammalian cells.

If these reports are true then nature has been unkind. For in good weather, at ground level, there are more positive ions than negative ions. Hot and dry weather increase the positive ions, making people feel uncomfortable. Altered behavior of cattle before a storm is supposed to be due to a rapid buildup of positive ions. Negative ions increase the most when large amounts of water strike the air. The sweet smelling air just after a thunderstorm is due to this effect.

A panel of physicians and meteorologists have studied the effects of weather, seasons, climate, and atmospheric conditions on human health, and their report was issued by the World Meteorological Organization of the U. N. It contains some strange statistical correlations and speculations.

Changes in the atmospheric electrical fields during thunderstorms cause traffic accidents because of slow driver-reaction time. These atmospheric conditions may also precipitate an 11% increase in births and 20% in deaths.

Certain diseases, according to these same biometeorologists, are influenced by weather changes. Asthmatic attacks are not common when the barometric pressure is high or there is fog, but are increased when the pressure is low and there is a sudden cooling of the air. Glaucoma attacks, due to increased pressure in the eye, occur more frequently on very hot or very cold days. Epileptic seizures are brought on by rapid changes in light intensity. Stomach ulcer perforations are more common in the spring and fall, especially during extreme alterations in air movements.

The eyes, nose, throat, lungs, skin, and nervous system are the chief parts of the body which react to weather changes say these scientists. Climatic stress or disease may weaken temperature-control mechanisms in the body and thereby produce drug reactions. They point out that digitalis is more dangerous when the atmospheric temperature rises. Stimulating drugs (analeptics) increase in toxicity as the temperature falls. Strychinine is more effective in cold weather.

Furthermore they assert marked weather changes are bad for health but quiet air masses are beneficial. Hot air masses preceding the influx of cold air, low barometric pressures, and intermediate zones between high and low pressures are inimical to health. The lee sides of high mountains are protective.

We have alluded to electromagnetism in the atmosphere and its influence on man. How about man also being an electromagnetic entity? All cells contain a minute charge of electricity. David Cohn of MIT and Louis Chandler of Rutgers University have studied this phenomenon. They point out that weak magnetic fields are produced in living creatures by ion currents. Examples are the brain wave (Alpha rhythm) currents which give rise to part of the electroencephalogram recording, the electrical currents arising from voluntary muscular activity, and heart currents which produce the electrocardiogram. Cohn and Chandler in studying the heart, found that there is a cardiac magnet field appearing outside the body. Further investigations may result in discovering values not available in surface electrocardiography. Cohn also showed that there exists weak magnetic fields surrounding the head and outside the scalp.

Are these electromagnetic shells subject to alteration by external as well as internal factors? Intrinsic factors would be disease and drugs. External factors would be our cosmos, the earth's electromagnetic atmosphere, and its gravitational force. The earth is a giant floating magnet. The living being is a microcosmic magnet.

There is a form of therapy known as electrosleep. It was begun in Russia over 20 years ago and in Germany 10 years ago. In this treatment a pair of electrodes are placed over the eyes and another pair behind the ears. A weak current flows between these electrodes into the brain. There are about 300 centers for electrosleep therapy in Russia and hundreds of articles have appeared in Russian literature describing its use in conditions ranging from asthma to schizophrenia.

There has been some work done in this country, but electrotherapy has been associated with quackery in the past. Recognized therapy has been electroshock, long and short wave diathermy, ultra sonics, and more recently pulsed electrotherapy.

Psychiatrist Ronald Koegler has reported improvement in his patients with sleep problems after electrosleep therapy. Most of these patients were chronic insomniacs or depressives. He reports that when the current is first turned on over the eyes there is a temporary pricking sensation followed by the patients seeing black and white. Then color sensations appear. This phenomenon has been compared to mild LSD effects.

Other physicians express their opinion on this modality. Norman Wulfsohn, anesthesiologist of the University of Texas Medical School, believes that electrosleep has potential in treating insomnia, anxiety neuroses, and depression. Norman Post tried electrosleep in stroke patients and notes there is some reduction in the spasticity of the limbs, more so in the arms than legs. Patient outlook and sleep also improve. Post prefers the term "transcerebral electrotherapy" to electrosleep because all patients do not fall asleep. Internist Bernard Straus tested more than 100 patients and says that electrosleep is as effective as phenobarbital in ordinary sleep producing doses.

Anatomist Carmine Clemente of UCLA, a sleep researchist, found that electrostimulation of the basal forebrain would put an animal to sleep within seconds. This action inhibits the transmission of nerve impulses in the brain stem and upper spinal cord. Clemente feels that the popular theory on sleep, that it is due to a slowdown or fatigue of activity in the reticular part of the brain is wrong. He believes that the brain structures that cause sleep may be different than those which control wakefulness.

Some American researchers are against electrosleep, claiming that too much current must be used to get through in some patients. This causes skin burns, increased heart rate, rise in blood pressure, and spasticity of muscles.

The Russians emphatically state that this therapy has a healing effect on stomach ulcers. Larson, Reigel, and Sances, investigators at Marquette University, found that in monkeys electrosleep markedly cuts down stomach acid secretion.

German reports state that electrosleep is effective in heroin addiction therapy. The individual is first taken off heroin and put on methadone. Then in due course he is given electrosleep to kick the methadone habit.

We are still in the preliminary period of this investigation. The brain is partly an electric organ, and perhaps we need special types of currents, exact places to apply them, and perhaps coordination with circadian rhythms (which has not been done to date) to secure the best therapeutic results.

Physicist Erwin Saxl, in experiments with a torsion pendulum rotating through a fixed path both clockwise and counterclockwise and with its movements recorded electronically, noted a periodicity in the times required to perform this function. There was a daily diurnal rhythm and also seasonal variations.

During the eclipse of March 7, 1970, he observed significant variations in the timing during the phenomenon as well as in the hours preceding and following the event. Between the onset of the eclipse and its midpoint there was a steady increase in timing. After the midpoint the timing decreased suddenly, and then leveled off to greater values than those seen before the eclipse. Furthermore, preceding the eclipse, there was a periodic variation in the timing. This strange periodicity was seen again two weeks later at the same hours of the day, although the sun and moon were on opposite sides of the earth. This time the readings were somewhat higher.

Saxl's work is a great breakthrough in science, showing that the classical gravitational theory held for many years needs to be modified to interpret these newly found facts.

This scientist has noted, during his experiments with the torsion pendulum over the years at Harvard, Massachusetts, a wavelike repetition of periodicity which cannot be explained, predicted, or recorded on the basis of the classical gravitational theory. For Saxl's pendulum moves perpendicularly to the earth's gravity vector unlike the instruments which are quasistationary and support the old theory of gravity. As a result of these observations we see that the force of the earth's gravity is also periodic, and that we live in and are a part of a rhythmic universe.

Chapter Twenty

POLLUTION

POLLUTION IS THE PRESENCE in the air, water, or on the earth of substances injurious to man's environment, health, and welfare. While many of these things are the products of man's culture and are human pollutants, others are natural pollutants contributed by natural phenomena.

From the cosmos comes radiation which can damage or kill individuals. Examples of this are the x-rays, ultraviolet, and infrared rays hurled into our atmosphere by the convulsions of the sun.

Upheavals from the earth, in the form of volcanic eruptions, spew out large masses of hot lava, noxious fumes, and gases into the atmosphere. Earthquakes precipitated by our quivering planet split open the ground, letting gases escape into our atmosphere. Hurricane and sandstorms temporarily pollute our environment with salt spray or sand respectively.

Natural airborne pollutants that cause disease are: dusts, pollens from trees, grasses, and weeds; bacteria, viruses, and fungi; smuts and rusts from diseased plants; substances such as feathers, animal hairs and danders, certain flowers and plants, insects and mites.

All living matter on this earth exists in a narrow layer known as the biosphere. This is a region in which water is adequately present, sunlight is received in sufficient quantities, and there are interfaces between land, water, and the gaseous atmosphre. More specifically it means the land surface with its thin topsoil, the upper regions of lakes, rivers, and the oceans, and the atmosphere with specific gases which will support life forms.

All life's energy comes from the sun. It can only enter living systems through photosynthesis performed by chlorophyll containing organisms such as purple and green bacteria, blue-green algae, the phytoplankton of lakes and seas, and higher plants. In this process sunlight and chlorophyll convert carbon dioxide, water, and salts to organic compounds, while oxygen is released as a spinoff. In turn, living and dead organisms are oxidized to produce carbon dioxide and so the cycle continues.

In addition to carbon, nitrogen, oxygen, and hydrogen, living beings need a variety of chemicals. The presence or lack of such elements determine how much life can be sustained in a particular locality. Phosphorus is perhaps the most limiting chemical. If the biosphere is to be sustained, the essential substances must revert back again for reuse so that the cycle may continue.

A new situation is disrupting this ancient, finely-balanced rhythm. Man has unwittingly introduced the unnatural cycling of harmful elements and compounds such as lead, mercury, insecticides, and defoliants. The injurious effect of these and other substances on living light-synthesizing forms needs thorough investigation and strong measures to stop it.

The sun's energy, which is absorbed by the earth, is eventually radiated back into space. This cycle seems to work with a definite precision. In the interim between radiation and reradiation, the circulation of the atmosphere and the movements of the oceans distribute the energy over the surface of the planet. Natural or unnatural changes started by man may alter the stability of this feedback. Cloud cover or increased dust pollution at extremely high altitudes may reflect back more radiation, leaving less available for heating the earth. Slowly increasing carbon dioxide levels in our atmosphere increase heat retention.

The modern biosphere did not simply happen. It began about three billion years ago, when very simple organisms came into existence which could exist on organic matter. To survive they had to live at sufficient depths in water or sediments to avoid the deadly ultraviolet rays coming through the primitive atmosphere. A billion years later new forms appeared which released oxygen into an environment completely devoid of this gas. The more primitive forms then died out, for oxygen was poisonous to them.

With the continual production of oxygen by photosynthesizing cells over hundreds of millions of years, oxygen increased gradually, building up into an aerial layer able to screen out the sun's destructive rays. About 400 million years ago the land became available for the growth and utilization by oxygen-consuming living systems. Evolution produced many varieties of plants and animals which helped to build and stabilize the modern biosphere we recognize today.

While agriculture, during this century, has been highly productive, the use of fertilizers, herbicides, and pesticides has adversely affected ecological systems far away from the source of application. Restraints are now being considered or applied by various countries.

Despite previous impressions, the oceans are not an unlimited source of food for the human race. According to Ryther, the potential yearly yield of fish will be no greater than 100 million tons. In 1967, the total catch was a little over 60 million tons. For the past 25 years it has been increasing annually at about 8%, and, based upon these calculations, the fishing industry can expand for about a decade. Not taken into account, of course, is the effect of pollution which may drastically alter these figures. For even now, fish hauls are being condemned because they contain dangerous amounts of toxic substances. So it becomes quite obvious that the oceans cannot support the expanding human population.

Local heat pollution raises the water temperature of streams, rivers, and lakes, and destroys the food supply needed by edible fish. Decay follows, and as it increases, oxygen disappears from the water killing the fish. The life forms still surviving in the water shift from an aerobic (oxygenated) to an anerobic (non-oxygenated) form. Consequently, organic matter builds up in the water with production of poisonous gases such as methane and hydrogen sufide.

In the last 100 years, the increased exploitation of fossil fuels such as coal, natural gas, and oil, have produced a 10% increase in carbon dioxide levels in the air, along with an increased photosynthesis by plants. There has also been a rise in temperature, but more recently a decline. This lower temperature will reduce periods of favorable vegetation growth. Toxic wastes, in addition, will affect the ecological systems unfavorably.

The major ecological systems, called ecosystems, of our planet are being reduced by the building of cities, roads, and increased agricultural deployment. The toxic products from the man dominated areas are gradually destroying the remaining ecosystems.

Another alarming happening is the increasing of fine particles in the atmosphere such as sulfates, nitrates, and hydrocarbons. They both reflect and absorb solar radiation. What the long range results on temperature will be, we do not know.

In the stratosphere we are encountering another problem. High flying planes are introducing fine particles of carbon dioxide and water vapor. The former will probably have no effect, but the doubling of fine particles and an increase of about 10 percent in water vapor may make a difference by raising the temperature of the stratosphere and increasing cloudiness.

Back here on earth, we have to wrestle with the pesticide problem. While one chemical may get rid of a particular pest, its toxicity may kill the predators of a locality, allowing new pests to proliferate. So we exchange one agonizing problem for another. Toxic pesticides such as DDT create a special problem for they do not disintegrate but persist indefinitely in the tissues of man and animals.

Oil has many valuable industrial uses. But when oil is spilled into the oceans at the rate of one and a half million tons a year and when several times as much is dumped or lost on the ground, then we have a mounting defilement of our environment. Means and methods must be found for recycling of used oil instead of polluting our land and seas.

Overfertilization of our lakes, springs and rivers, known as eutrophication, is caused by nitrates and phosphorus. These substances come from sewage and the runoffs from fertilized crops. Detergents are now being studied and phosphorus is being deleted from such products. It is essential that there be recycling and reclaimation of sewage and other runoffs to stop this defilement of our waters.

Mercury is valuable in industry and in the medical profession. It is used in making thermometers, batteries, lamps, electrical appliances, pesticides, paper production, antiseptic preparations, and formerly as a cathartic and in the treatment of syphilis. Mercury, as a pollutant, has been coming from industrial plants, and eventually ending up at the bottom of lakes, streams and oceans. These locales were once considered safe havens to dispose of this material. However, bacteria in the mud convert inorganic harmless mercury into organic dimethyl mercury in order to purge their own environment. The compound then enters the marine food chain and ends up in our edible fish and eventually in us. Mercury can damage the kidney, brain, liver and other organs. It can severely incapacitate or kill.

Nitrates stimulate the algae in water to proliferate at a fast rate. The massive overpopulation depletes the oxygen and fish soon asphyxiate. Unless fertilizers and nitrogenous wastes are prudently managed, our fresh water supplies from rivers and lakes becomes polluted. The problem of such disposal magnifies because of the increasing human and animal population. Waste nitrate products should be recycled, but efficient methods are yet to be devised.

Throughout man's history, his numbers were regulated by the food supply available. For millions of years, and we still do not know how many, man got his food by being a predator, scavenger, or by eating vegetation. Under these conditions, the biosphere could support no more than 10 million humans. When man learned to domesticate animals and plants, about 10,000 years ago, he began to alter the biosphere to his own benefit. With increased food supply, more humans were able to survive. The population has been increasing so fast in this century that the biosphere is in danger of collapsing.

Today, agriculture has taken over about 3 billion acres of land that were formerly grasslands or forests, or about 1/10th of the earth's total land area. About 2/3rds of this total is planted with cereal grains. Genetics have improved the quality of grains, crops, and animals. Mechanization, along with fertilization and chemical control of weeds and pests, has increased food output, but unfortunately disturbed the ecosystems of the biosphere.

In heavy populated countries like India and China, large forest areas have been stripped away. Consequently wood is scarce and cow dung is used for fuel. Livestock provides power for haulage, as well as producng food and fuel. The number of animals increases with the population, and they despoil further, the countryside of grass. With the loss of this natural cover, erosion sets in. The soil blows into the atmosphere or washes away with the rains and ends up in the seas. The land becomes a wasteland as in India. North Africa was once the granary of the Roman Empire. Today it is a desert or near desert. In the USA we had our "dust bowl" in the 1930's but luckily with planning we reclaimed it. Recently, in the USSR, 100 million acres of plowed land with inadequate rainfall became ruined. Soil erosion is one of the most pressing problems threatening the future of our biosphere, especially in Asia, the Middle East, North Africa, and Central America.

Today one seventh of the earth's land surface is desert. Together, with semi-desert regions, we find that three tenths of the planet's land surface is denuded. This is equal to an area 4½ times the size of the entire United States. For lack of water these regions cannot produce food. Modern irrigation is not making appreciable gains in these lands, for deserts in many areas are growing faster than they can be reclaimed by modern technology. In Africa, pasture lands are being rapidly depleted, and deserts are growing at the rate of 247,000 acres a year. It is reported that in some regions the desert is advancing 30 miles a year, which certainly seems fantastic if true.

Scientists are considering schemes to reclaim the deserts. A source of usable water must be found, along with a stable and intelligent government, a good economic system, and an educated citizenry. The most basic problem is still the lack of water and topsoil.

There are plans to change the world's weather patterns. One involves the use of carbon to blacken the Artic ice so as to retain more solar energy. With more heat the region might become inhabitable with larger populations. Another idea is to dam the Bering Straight and pump icy Artic water into the Pacific Ocean to improve the weather in this climate. One novel design to change world weather is to create a five mile thick ice cloud over the Arctic by exploding 10 hydrogen bombs which would generate a steam cloud that would quickly freeze. A plan to blast holes through the Sierra Nevada Mountains would allow moist Pacific air to pour rain into the Nevada desert and make it bloom. There are many other grandiose schemes. Whether they will work as their planners dream or whether they would produce catastrophic results is not known.

Even irrigation brings problems. It raises the water table, which may then inhibit the growth of plant roots by water logging. This action also results in the soil becoming saline, as the rising water evaporates through it leaving the dissolved salts. West Pakistan encountered this problem after using the water of the Indus river for irrigation for about a century. American know-how overcame the situation by drilling tube wells to lower the water table. The ground water was then tapped for intensive irrigation and discharged on the surface to get rid of the salts. However, in the past, such lands were abandoned, leading to the decline and disappearance of civilizations in the Middle East. Irrigation has brought a great increase in the disease known as schistosomiasis in both Africa and Asia and afflicts about 250 million people. This is discussed in the chapter on parasitic diseases.

The production of energy from fossil fuels today is enormous, and it affects the environment by creating large amounts of carbon dioxide. The five most common pollutants accompanying it are carbon monoxide, sulfur oxides, hydrocarbons, nitrogen oxides, and solid particles. Airborne lead, from the combustion of leaded gasoline, is another serious contaminant. The major sources of fouling of the air are automobiles, industry, power plants, incinerators, home heating units, and garbage and trash disposals.

This unclean air ruins paint, corrodes buildings and automobiles, splotches laundry, destroys vegetation, trees, and crops, and affects the health of humans and animals. It is blamed for an increase in diseases such as strokes, coronary heart attacks, emphysema, bronchitis, cirrhosis of the liver, arthritis, eye and nasal disorders, neuroses, psychoses, and cancer. The hydrocarbons and nitrous oxides help to form smog, a very irritating form of air pollution.

The dirty air indirectly affects surface water, because the rains carry the contaminants down from the atmosphere. In addition, the dispersal of waste water from power plants adds to the defilement. Fossil fuels will eventually be exhausted, just when is not known precisely. Some scientists believe they will disappear by the 23rd century, and that petroleum will run out within 75 years.

An important source of pollution is solid wastes. An improved efficiency of cycling is necessary to combat the problem. This task must succeed, not only to prevent our depletion of shrinking natural resources, but also to stop contaminating the biosphere. The quantity of wastes now being produced are astronomical. It has been estimated that each American is responsible for about a ton of waste each year. One third of this is packaged materials. In 1968 every American was supposed to have thrown away 300 cans, 150 bottles, and 300 pounds of paper. Each year disposable items are increasing and this trend must be reversed. Proper recycling would provide raw materials for steel, aluminum, glass and the plastics industries.

A number of researchers claim that the air in our homes is just as polluted as outside air, and in many cases it is even worse. Listed among the sources producing contamination are:

gas stoves	hair and other aerosol sprays
gas and hot air furnaces	stain solvents
insecticides	sponge rubber furniture and beddings
smoking	house dusts
paint products	odors
deodorants	emanations
disinfectants	particulate matter from raw or cooked food
pastics	cleaning and scouring agents
waxes	bacteria
viruses	molds

Also potentially damaging are microwave ovens and x-ray radiation from TV sets. These facts lead one to wonder whether home is the safest place after all.

Once, and it now seems a long time ago, the rivers of this country contained pure water, good wholesome fish and shellfish. Today pure water is a rarity. Fish and shellfish, that have not been killed off, are heavily polluted. Rivers are now running foul with human excrement, garbage, and industrial poisons. People drinking this water are being infected with lethal diarrhea-producing microbes such as salmonella and shigella. Fish and shellfish taken and eaten from these waters produce gastrointestinal diseases and even death. They must be thoroughly cooked to destroy the microorganisms they contain. Hepatitis and typhoid fever have occurred from the consumption of polluted water and its food offerings.

Pesticides such as DDT, endrin, aldrin, dieldrin, parathion, malathion, chlordane, and lindane have proven to be of great value in agriculture, gardening, and for household use. However, their worldwide distribution and their harmful effect on living forms other than pests is now well apparent. Marine life is being adversely affected, sometimes with catastrophic destruction of fish populations in streams, lakes, and rivers. The bird population is also in danger of extinction.

It is said that the human body is so contaminated with DDT, that it could never pass the standards set for animal meats fit for human consumption. Human milk contains more DDT than cow's milk. Mother's milk was once considered the safest food for infants.

Pesticide usage is constantly increasing. It is no longer possible to escape its effects. Even if one only consumes organically grown foods, he still breathes, drinks, and eats fish and meats contaminated with chemicals. There have even been many reports in the USA of people dying from eating foods poisoned with pesticides.

Evidence is accumulating that some pesticides cause sexual impotency in men. Reports are not cumulative, as yet, on sterility effects. But this has been noticed in animals where reproduction is falling off and certain species are faced with extinction. There is little reason to assume that man may not be similarly afflicted. Pesticides cause cancer in animals, and it may be a factor in humans also.

Today there is much talk about people pollution. The unrestricted propagation of human beings must cease sooner or later, preferably sooner. This world can only support a limited number of individuals, because the supplies of food and fresh water are also limited.

In prehistoric times, possibly 10 million humans existed. At about the time of the Roman Empire this number had increased to about 100 million souls. In this century the population has jumped by billions, the greatest increase in the history of man.

Medical advancements and scientific technology are responsible for this dilemma. Before man upset nature's balance, there was an ecological equilibrium. Infectious disease was a powerful weapon in controlling population and this factor was mainly upset during this century.

Contraception is being advanced in many countries to halt excessive births. While there is opposition by some religious groups, the realities of the situation must be faced. The sordid facts of overpopulation with its poverty, squalor, malnutrition, disease, and crime must be faced. The more people we have the more food and fresh water is needed, and more pollution of the environment follows. The institution of legal abortion in various states and nations is another effort to cut down excessive and unwanted births, and this, too, meets with opposition. When not permitted, illegal abortion with all its horrors continues. People are not always rational when they must come to grips with unpleasant and undesirable situations.

If we are fortunate to escape disability, disease, or death by pollution of our water, air, and food, another danger lurks for us. This peril comes from the deliberate introduction of chemical additives in our foods and water.

Because competition is sharp in the food industry, processors attempt to make their products as appealing as possible. Foods are preserved for long life on the shelves, colored for eye appeal, sweetened for taste desirability, and attractively packaged. But this is not all. Foods are cured, salted, emulsified and stabilized, polished, bleached, gassed to ripen, degermed, defatted, and sprayed. Animal foods receive special treatment with sex hormones, antibiotics, tranquilizers, disinfectants, antispoilants, enzymes, desiccants, and sex sterilants.

If one reads the list of chemicals on the labels of food products, he is truly amazed. Some of these chemicals are toxic, some carcinogenic or suspected of being so, and the action of many is actually unknown. In addition to these dangers, natural substances in foods are destroyed, decreased, or altered in some fashion. This is especially true of vitamins. A sampling of some commercial foods will be given.

Mostly all canned juices contain benzoic acid for preservation. They may also include the antifoaming agent, dimethyl polysiloxane, which is a mild depressant. Dyes to color the fruit and synthetic flavoring agents, whose safety is not fully known, are added to the concoction along with a sweetening substance such as sugar or saccharin.

Now let's look at the old staff of life, the ubiquitous bread. The seed, when planted, was treated with mercury bichloride. As it grew it was sprayed with toxic insecticides and also pesticides. When ground eventually into flour, the cereal grain was bleached with agene, now mostly discarded as being very dangerous, or chlorine dioxide which is far from innocuous. Then a dough conditioner, ammonium chloride, is added. To make the bread feel soft and fresh, polyoxyethylene, which irritates the skin, is added. Then an antioxidant, ditertiary-butylpara-cresol, is mixed in along with bromate to improve the quality of the flour. Both of these chemicals are toxic. Yellow dyes may be added, if the manufacturers wish to fool the public into believing a lot of eggs and butter has been used. Finally, calcium propionate is thrown in to prevent molding of the bread. This chemical mixture is the twentieth century alchemist's creation of what constitutes good wholesome bread.

Succulent roast beef comes from cattle which are fed corn and hay sprayed with pesticides and fed the synthetic female hormone stilbestrol. This chemical fattens the cattle. Antibiotics are also given to the animals to increase their weight. Stilbestrol is said to destroy vitamin B & E. It is believed to have some carcinogenic affect. We ingest it every time we eat beef, veal, chicken, turkey, and ham.

Our old favorite desert, ice cream, has not escaped the food alchemists either. It was originally made of cream, eggs, fruit flavoring, and sugar. But this was a long time ago. Now it contains a stabilizer and expander, known as carboxymethylcellulose, to make the volume of ice cream seem much larger. Monoglycerides, diglycerides, artificial fats, and chemicals are employed to emulsify the preparation into a smooth creamy texture. Then comes artificial flavors and colorings to make it tasty and eye appealing, and who knows what else?

While old fashioned sweet cream, whether eaten as is or whipped, is high in cholesterol, it is far less harmful than the various substitute toppings on the market. They contain many chemicals such as hydrogenated vegetable oil, sodium phosphate, mono and diglycerides, sodium caseinate, polyoxyethylene, cellulose gum, calcium chloride, starch, coconut oil, corn syrup, vanilla flavor, and salt, all charged with nitrous oxide and carbon dioxide gas in an aerosol can.

Butter contains nordihydroguairatic acid which prevents rancidity, a chemical barred by Canadian authorities but condoned in the USA. Diacetyl is also inserted to provide a butter smelling and flavoring agent. Yellow dyes are added to provide color and most of them are coal tar derivatives. Also present are substances the cows have ingested such as insecticides, pesticides, antibiotics, and hormones.

To stop salt from sticking and to keep it free flowing, potassium iodide, calcium hydroxide (caustic soda) and calcium silicate are added.

The chemicalization of our food is staggering to comprehend. Experts state that about 2,000 chemicals are deliberately added to foods, and about 1500 additives end up in products during processing or packaging. There are 30 categories of additives, and the largest group is the 1200 flavoring agents. Frequently a mixture of many agents is needed to blend the required flavor. Other major categories are preservatives, vitamins, stabilizers, emulsifiers, and minerals.

About 1500 new food products come on the market each year such as frozen foods and quickly-prepared meat dishes which are heavily chemicalized. They are easily prepared and have long shelf life.

Among new additions already out or being prepared, are synthetic butter-flavored salt for popcorn, a synthetic pepper flavor, synthetic coffee and fresh-baked-bread flavors. The food industry is using vegetable protein, like soybean, to create artificial foods such as bacon, ground beef, or scallops. To complete the illusion flavors, colors, stabilizers, preservatives, and other necessary chemicals are included.

Even now the food industry is planning to produce artificial fruits and vegetables by using additives which will give the synthetic preparation the textural properties of common fruits and vegetables. How far shall we stray from nature and still survive?

The organic farmers use natural fertilizers such as compost made up of rotting vegetation, cattle or other manure, unconsumed food, and any other organic material available. On this material they pile thick mulches of grass clippings or straw to crowd out weeds and retain moisture. No chemicals are used at all. The food grown under these conditions is far superior to that sold in supermarkets.

This technique closely approximates natural methods of fertilization. For, in the normal course of events, nature gives back to the soil that which she removed. Natural fertilizer is composed of unused pollens and the rotting of dead leaves, branches, and trees. To this decomposition is added that of decaying vegetation and animals, and also animal excreta. Certain soil bacteria and fungi break down these substances for recycling. Nitrogen-fixing soil bacteria convert the nitrogen of the air into nitrate nutrients for plant use. Nature adds some airborne elements such as nitrates generated in the atmosphere by electrical storms, meteor and space dust, and nutrients generated in the atmosphere by floating life forms.

To the argument that it is prohibitive to compost a large field, Rodale answers with the statement that one such application will

Drugs, Demons, Doctors, and Disease

outlast many doses of artificial chemical fertilizers. A good shower of rain will wash away phosphates applied to the soil, while compost may stay in the soil for years. Depletion of the soil depletes soil bacteria and thereby prevents digestion of soil nutrients. Sick soil breeds sick plants. The answer is not to apply more chemicals and toxic substances, but to return to the ways of nature and replenish the earth.

Finally there is noise pollution. Too much decible stimulation is taking a heavy toll of human health, and some consider it as bad as smog or dirty water. The price is exacted, say the experts, in heart attacks, high blood pressure, damage to unborn babies, nervous disorders, tensions and irritability, and loss of hearing.

The noise level of modern life has increased continually. Rock music, sonic booms, constant ground and air traffic sounds, radio and TV stimulation, all add their increments to this situation. It has become a very noisy world. Attempts are being made to try to lower the disagreeable sound assaults on people.

In summing up, we find that modern life is not simple, but very complex. Individuals are perplexed by environmental problems; the accident of birth into a particular color, race, religion, and economic level; the dirty, noisy, overcrowded, poverty stricken, and crime ridden cities; the agony of public and private transportation; poor public schools which are deteriorating and still offering instruction irrelevant to today's living. If all this is not enough there is still more. We have international and racial tensions, wars, and a nuclear race. We have mounting inflation, higher and higher taxes, and a debt-financed country. Youth has turned on to hallucenogenic drugs, rebelling against what they call a tobacco-alcoholic hangup by their elders. Many of the elders, to be part of the scene, have also turned on to hallucenogenics.

Some say communism is the answer, others capitalism, a few revert to communal experiments which were often tried in the past and turned out to be failures. There are prophets who shout that the world should repent and turn back to God and religion. Many want science to provide the answers. There are stoics who do their best and do not expect too much. Others are hedonists, living only for today.

When we add to this confusion such additional items as pollution, food additives, a government unable or unwilling to grapple with these problems, we do not see too much hope for optimism at this time. However, if we go back and study history, we cannot find any time when there were no serious problems confronting man. Yet he has managed to survive, muddle through, and reach high levels of cultural and technological science, while retaining a spiritual outlook on his earthly presence. The final story of man has not yet been written.